LEAVING

Youth suicide: the horror, the heartbreak, the hope

EARLY

BRONWYN DONAGHY

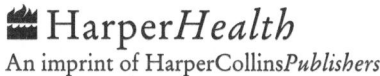
Harper*Health*
An imprint of HarperCollins*Publishers*

Harper*Health*

An imprint of HarperCollins*Publishers*, Australia

First published in Australia in 1997
Reprinted in 1997, 1998, 1999, 2000, 2001
by HarperCollins*Publishers* Pty Limited
ABN 36 009 913 517
A member of the HarperCollins*Publishers* (Australia) Pty Limited Group
www.harpercollins.com.au

Published in association with the NSW Centre for the Advancement of Adolescent
health at the New Children's Hospital, Westmead. A proportion of the royalties of
this book will go to the Centre to help further their goal of promoting and
improving the health and well-being of Australian adolescents and their families.

HarperCollins*Publishers*
25 Ryde Road, Pymble, Sydney NSW 2073, Australia
31 View Road, Glenfield, Auckland 10, New Zealand

National Library of Australia Cataloguing-in-Publication data:

Donaghy, Bronwyn, 1948– .
   Leaving early: youth suicide – the horror, the heartbreak, the hope.
   Includes index.
   ISBN 0 7322 5781 6.
   1. Youth – Australia – Suicidal behavior. 2. Youth –
   Australia – Suicidal behavior – Case studies. 3. Suicide –
   Australia – Prevention. I. Title.
362.280835.

Permission to use the photographs of Collin Schultz and Jason Connor on the cover
has been kindly granted by their families. Additional photography by Paula Marchant.

Excerpts from *The Past, Civilisation* and *Song of Hope* by Oodgeroo of the tribe
Noonuccal (formerly known as Kath Walker) are from *My People*, third edition,
1990 by Jacaranda Press, Reprinted with permission.

Printed and bound in Australia by Griffin Press on 79gsm Bulky Paperback White

10 9 8 7 6   01 02 03 04

CONTENTS

Part three

ABOUT THE AUTHOR

Bronwyn Donaghy is the author of the best-selling *Anna's Story*, which explored adolescent drug abuse, and has sold over 70,000 copies. For two decades Bronwyn has specialised in writing about issues that affect families, and her articles and columns have appeared in the *Sydney Morning Herald*, *Australia's Parents* magazine, *New Woman*, *Family Circle* and many other publications. Her parenting survival guide *Keeping Mum* was published in 1997.

A MESSAGE FROM PROFESSOR BEVERLEY RAPHAEL
Director, Centre for Mental Health
New South Wales Health Department

'This book offers compassionate and sensitive insights into the human lives and human suffering surrounding youth suicide. No other work gives such honest and painful accounts of the lives of young people and their families through these tragic experiences. This book is a tribute, a testimony and a hope. By sharing their lives these families have helped us to see this problem in sharp relief. By her concerned depiction of the issues Bronwyn Donaghy not only offers insights, but also shows hopeful ways forward, and the possibility of mastering the challenges of youth suicide. It is a book for care, for compassion, for strengthening our concern and for a chance to make things better.'

To Frankie

My husband, my friend

ALSO BY BRONWYN DONAGHY

2½ Wishes (a novel for children)
Anna's Story
Keeping Mum
Unzipped

Foreword

The youth suicide rate in this country is among the highest in the Western world. There would be few Australians, regardless of age, who do not know at least something about this problem; whether it be through media reporting, clinical involvement, academic debate or government policy making. And for far too many young people, their families and friends the connection with the issue is agonisingly personal and devastatingly sad.

Leaving Early courageously explores the phenomenon of adolescent and young adult suicide, its complex meanings and life-shattering realities. During the months of research and writing involved in its creation, I was privileged to watch Bronwyn Donaghy's creative struggle with a thousand questions: what to include, who to consult, what to emphasise, how to proceed. As with her earlier book, *Anna's Story*, the outcome is an outstanding achievement – a uniquely interwoven text encompassing true stories, expert commentary, current facts and heart-rending reflections. The people who have shared their grief are present in the full richness of their characters – for their generosity of spirit, we are deeply grateful. And throughout it all, the author's own caring and concerned voice is clearly heard.

Many important messages resonate throughout these pages, from the disturbing prevalence of depression among young people to the frequent failings of our health system in the face of emotional crisis, from the special plight of Aboriginal and rural youth to the valued support of self-help groups and the importance of hope.

Leaving Early is the first in a series of books, authored by Bronwyn Donaghy, which tackle some of the pressing contemporary issues in adolescent health. It represents a collaboration involving HarperCollins*Publishers* and the NSW Centre for the Advancement of Adolescent Health at the New Children's Hospital, Sydney.

I sincerely commend this book to you and urge you to share it with others.

Clinical Associate Professor David Bennett AO MBBS FRACP

Head, Department of Adolescent Medicine

The New Children's Hospital and Westmead Hospital and Community Services

Westmead, New South Wales

Author's acknowledgments

When I was asked to write a book on youth suicide my immediate reaction was one of horror. How could I write about a subject as sad as this? How could anyone?

Then I met some of the families of the young people concerned and I thought: how could I not?

It has taken enormous courage for Jan and Ron Schultz, Peter and Lee Connor, and the sisters, brothers and friends of Collin, Jason and the girl I have called Maz, to tell their stories.

They have done so in the hope that, at best, other young lives may be saved and, at least, their words might go a little way towards reducing the stigma of suicide, while bringing some comfort to those who are suffering from similar tragic loss.

I would like to thank them and all the other people who told me their stories during the writing of this book, including Ruth Anderson and Ron McLean who prepared written as well as verbal contributions.

I am particularly grateful to Tony Humphrey, from Club Speranza, and Gail Kilby, from the Rose Foundation, who took so much time, trouble and care to put me in touch with the bereaved families.

The idea for *Leaving Early* was suggested by Associate Professor David Bennett, Director of the NSW Centre for the Advancement of Adolescent Health at the New Children's Hospital, Westmead. I appreciate the guidance provided by Dr Bennett and by the Centre Coordinator, Dr Michael Reed throughout this project.

I am indebted to many other professional people who assisted me with the research. They include: Margaret Appleby and Dr Ray King from the Rose Foundation,

Professor Beverley Raphael, Julie Dunsmore, Barry Taylor, Richard Eckersley, Dr Michael Dudley, Dr Ernest Hunter, Dr George Patton, Dr Titia Sprague, Dr Sheila Clark, Jon Pfaff and John Anderson. Staff at the National Health and Medical Research Council and the Australian Bureau of Statistics were also very helpful.

Thank you, too, to my editors, Robin Freeman, Carolyn Leslie and Jennie Orchard for their thoughtful encouragement.

The Schultz family and their son's friends chose to use their real names in this book. The Connor family used real first names and a fictional surname. The exception is 'Lee' who, because of the personal nature of her own past history, elected to use a pseudonym. Where other pseudonyms have been used, these have been indicated with an asterisk.

All the people involved in Maz's (Marilyn's) story asked for complete anonymity for reasons which will become obvious. Some facts have been changed to protect their privacy. While Maz did keep a diary during her adolescence, and while I have used the device of a diary to tell her story, my main source of information was a series of taped interviews and written notes based on conversations, as it was with Collin's and Jason's stories.

Finally, I must thank my family for their support and understanding during what has been a sad and difficult project. I would like to add, however, that the people I have met during the writing of both *Leaving Early* and my earlier book, *Anna's Story*, have reinforced my belief that human kindness, compassion and decency are still alive and well in our society.

If only we could convince the kids.

Bronwyn Donaghy, September 1997

A glooming peace this morning with it brings;
The sun for sorrow will not show his head.
Go hence, to have more talk of these sad things.
From *Romeo and Juliet* by William Shakespeare

Prologue

The child was dancing on the edge of the shore, supervised by the rising sun.

He was small and skinny, a stick figure leaping on matchstick legs, escaping as the sea slung out each silver sheet, racing back up the beach while the folds of water slid up over the sand and flowed and billowed towards him.

Back and forth he ran, skipping down to the hem of each wave, scampering away, throwing back his curly head and laughing at his skill.

When his mother, in her gipsy dress, came down the beach to take him home, he squealed in protest and ran further into the water than he had dared to go before.

He didn't want to leave, he cried. Had she seen how fast he could run, how he whisked himself away from the big, wet water in the nick of time? Did she know how brave he was and how he could control the sea? Watch this! Watch this! Watch me!

The child danced at the edge of the world; he leapt and ran and jumped with the joy and promise of life.

He could do anything.

PART ONE

WHY?

Victoria, 1996: the train is late again. Another body on the tracks. A boy. Perfectly formed, olive-skinned, very smart, musical. Trains are efficient killing machines. Only the kids who leave early make them run late.

New South Wales, 1995: the ambulances are screaming again. Another body off the bridge. Another boy. Brilliant scholar, neat and sleek, funny. Gone early into the night-black water.

Queensland, 1994: a gun goes off. A body bleeds in the lush meadow grass. Another boy. Quiet, slow to speak, good with his hands. Leaving the pain for a grave on the hillside. Leaving early.

Western Australia, 1996: another mother's heart is broken. If only he could see her face. She throws her body over his, her baby, her big, beautiful child. The light of her life. Gone out.

New South Wales, 1997: the door swings open. A girl in the hospital bed, staring. Somebody came. Somebody cared. So she stayed. This time.

We can't keep reading. We shudder and turn away. This is not the sort of thing that could happen to us or ours; these were not your children, or mine.

We don't want to know. We don't want to think about it. Nobody wants to think about youth suicide.

Suicide is an intensely private act which creates unbearable public pain.

Anguished parents, heart-broken families, shocked and frightened friends, teachers, neighbours, colleagues, the newsagent, the butcher, the postman, the lady in the bank, even the people who read about it in the papers – in differing degrees, the act of suicide hurts us all.

Yet nobody wants to think or talk about it. Nobody is prepared to believe it can happen to them or theirs. Nobody can bear to believe that life can get *that* bad. Especially for young people.

But it does. In 1995, in Australia, at least 434 young men and women aged fifteen to twenty-four took their own lives. That's an average of eight a week. For every death, more than thirty other young people are trying to kill themselves.

For the bereaved families it seems that happiness on earth will never be possible again. Just going on with life – eating, sleeping, washing, working, driving, breathing – becomes agonisingly difficult under their burden of shocked pain and shocking guilt. For everyone concerned, there is horror, fear and denial.

The ripples from the rock that suicide hurls into the stream of the living spread far and wide, churning up love, loyalty and relationships, splashing the community with guilt and fear, seeping into future generations.

To take one's own life is an act terrible in its finality and terrifying in the questions it leaves behind – questions which can never be answered, giving rise to emotions too complex and contradictory to be truly understood. For those who are left there are no solutions. There is only shame, guilt, and the certainty that whatever contentment and security they may have achieved during their own lives has been destroyed forever by the conscious act of another person.

Families blame themselves. Friends blame themselves. Families and friends blame each other. Wives blame husbands. Husbands blame wives. Brothers blame sisters. Sisters and brothers blame lovers. And so on.

When a young person kills himself or herself, the unthinkable becomes a horrible reality. Intentional death on the brink of life threatens our own sense of continuity. Neither illness nor accident stopped this young heart from beating on. Almost always, the cause was sadness. And when young people are as seriously sad as this, the rest of us can't help but feel responsible.

All of life was ahead of them; all love, every opportunity, all beauty, pleasure, wonder and wisdom was theirs for the taking. Yet they flung back at the world the gifts life offered and walked away, closing the door forever behind them.

For families, the stigma is suffocating. In a society which has trouble dealing with death, death by suicide is shocking, frightening, unspeakable. Flowers. Do you send flowers? Church. Isn't suicide a sin? Where would the soul be? What will they say at the funeral? Casseroles. Do you take around a casserole? That would mean thinking of something to say to them. What *can* you say? There must have been something horribly wrong there somewhere. It makes you wonder. Drugs, probably. Surely not abuse? Was it the father's fault? Maybe the mother? Known them for years and no outward sign but maybe they didn't get on. Perhaps the kid was a bit of a horror; gave them a lot of trouble. Or a very bright child? Too much pressure on him? Discipline? Maybe they were too strict. You've got to be a bit broadminded in this day and age. But those poor parents. How must they feel? You thought that kid was made of stronger stuff. All those sporting trophies. And the way he did it ... it doesn't bear thinking about. Just don't think about it. It's none of your business really. Better to stay away. After all, what would you say?

You would say: 'I'm sorry. I can't begin to imagine how you feel. But I am truly sorry.'

The parents feel guilt, shame and rage. They feel the enormous frustration that comes with knowing that unlike death by accident or illness, death by suicide could have been prevented. There is no clinging to the belief that after all, there but for the grace of God go the rest of us. There is no relief in the thought that this could have happened to anyone.

They are convinced it could not.

But it can. In the words of community health educator, Gail Kilby: 'When I first started working in this area I was looking for reasons why this awful thing had happened to these particular families. I was looking for flaws, for faults in the way they ran their lives, for mistakes in the way they raised their children. I wanted to feel safe in the knowledge that it couldn't happen to me or mine.

'I discovered that there was no such guarantee. These people were just like me. These families were just like mine. Suicide can happen to anyone, anywhere, any time.'

The parents are overwhelmed with their sense of failure; ashamed that they were unable to prevent the death of their child.

I thought if there was a God up there He was saying: 'I gave you this precious gift, I put it in your care. And you destroyed it'.

Ruth Anderson, mother of Adam Kemp, 1976–1996

But they are angry too – furious that after giving their child years of love, bedtime stories, schooling, swimming lessons, nursing, sports training, clothing, a comfortable home, good food, great birthdays and complicated dental work, that child stopped on the threshold of adulthood and threw back the most precious gift of all – the gift of life. Took it, used it, rejected it and tossed it back in their faces.

With the suicide of one young person comes a new and previously unconsidered terror – that another child will follow suit. Or perhaps some other member of the family – or a close friend. The reality of suicide offers an option of escape which is too frightening to think about, but haunts their dreams in the quietest hours of the night and breaks into their thoughts in the noise of morning.

Friends share the guilt and outrage as well as the grief. Like the family, they wonder what they might have done to save their friend; girlfriends or boyfriends mourn for what might have been and what will never be again.

For the hopeless and disillusioned children of the street or the young unemployed men and women who live on the fringes of our communities, the sense of loss and abandonment is intensified.

Most of all, everyone wants to know *why*. What is happening to the world, when young men and women are choosing to cut their lives short rather than remain here?

Why is it the boys, and indeed the men, of Australia who are leaving life in the largest numbers? What is it about life at the turn of the twentieth century which is hurting boys and men so much?

Why are young people today so unhappy? After all, for centuries romances have been broken, jobs have been lost, wars have been fought, money has been scarce, loved ones have died or gone away. Families have been torn apart by changes other than divorce; the abuse of children is hardly a twentieth-century abomination.

It seems that in previous generations there were a lot more survival issues than there are now. Perhaps people who had to put so much energy into simply staying alive were less inclined to see death as a solution to their problems.

Then too, the predominantly Christian population of Australia used to believe not only that God would protect them in adversity, but that people who killed themselves went to hell. In an allegedly more enlightened era, we no longer expect our children to believe unquestionably in God, nor do we subscribe to religious horror stories – yet, in countries where that doctrine is still preached, the suicide rate is quite low.

Perhaps the most significant change that has come about in our society in the past thirty years is that religious and communal values have been eroded without being replaced with anything substantial in which young people can believe. In place of God, Queen and country, we encourage our young people to believe in themselves and we assist and applaud their acquisition of material things. Unfortunately, this sort of faith and success tends to disintegrate when life doesn't work out the way they would like it to do. Without some form of spiritual faith or anything concrete in the way of values and principles to conform to or even rage against, their hopelessness and disappointment revolves around themselves – sometimes with tragic consequences.

The main medical reason given for the increase in the number of youth suicides is depression. Previous generations have faced horrific diseases from rampant influenza to cholera and plague. But never before, it seems, have young people suffered so seriously from sadness.

Professor Beverley Raphael, the Director of the Centre for Mental Health in the New South Wales Health Department, calls it an epidemic of depression. 'We are living through a social phenomenon where there are increasingly high expectations of life yet there are far fewer opportunities to realise those expectations', she says.

'There is increased competitiveness, in education, in sport and everywhere else you can think of – we live in a highly competitive world where not everyone can win.

'Many parents have no idea how hard it is to be an adolescent today. It's hard to get a job, it's hard to get into university or into the right technical course. It's even harder for socially isolated teenagers or those from non-English speaking backgrounds or for young Aboriginal people.'

But most young people have no idea how hard it is to be the parent of an adolescent today, either. No matter how much we try, without the accepted values and discipline of the past, and without new guidelines to replace them, being a good mother or father has become a lonely, complicated and stressful business.

When our parents said we were not allowed to do something, almost every other parent in the street was saying it too. Now, if you are a caring parent who wants to know where your teenagers are going, insisting on rules and curfews, censoring the television they watch and advising them against taking drugs or having sex, there's no guarantee that the other parents in your suburb will be saying the same. These days, if you tell your kids they are expected to live by your rules while they are under your roof, it's acceptable for them to create enough aggravation to make everyone else in the house miserable for months. Or they can leave. One way or another.

Some parents today over-compensate their kids in an effort not to be as strict as their own parents were. And also, it must be said, for their own absence from home. But even the many parents who invest time and effort into supporting, advising and encouraging their children are not immune to the tragedy of youth suicide.

The current generation of young people seems to be much more cynical and street-smart than their parents; many young people make no secret of the fact that they feel alienated from the adult world.

'They want to be independent of you, but at the same time they get so frustrated when you don't have the answers,' said bereaved mother, Ruth Anderson. 'When they were little you fixed things for them but then they grow up and you can't solve their problems, you no longer have a bandaid that will stop them hurting. You may be just as confused as they are, but they can't cope with that.'

Some parents, who start out strongly, give up, worn down by the relentless struggle against peer pressure and the annihilating influence of the mass media. 'What can you do?' they ask each other. 'They think they know everything. You can talk but they never listen to a word you say anyway.'

Except that they do. They may rarely show it, but deep down in their multi-pierced ears they hear and they know you care about them. When parents stop talking it can be a sign to their adolescent and adult children that they have lost interest or given up on them.

Barry Taylor, a member of the Commonwealth youth suicide prevention advisory group, has visited centres in all states of Australia to examine proposed youth suicide prevention projects with a view to the allocation of government funding. He believes the adult literature and adult research into suicide doesn't apply to young people. 'We have to look at it from their perspective,' he said. 'We have to find out what it is about our society that is inducing young people to kill themselves.

'We are too inclined to look at immediate events – they've broken up with their girlfriend, they've lost their job, they've failed an exam – but these are things that happen to many young people without them killing themselves. So we say these kids must just be weak. In fact, there is almost always a background of events which has led to this act and this attitude.'

According to Barry Taylor, youth suicide prevention has to be about promoting good mental health. Life can be a very difficult journey and young people need to learn how to deal with the obstacles that will impede them along the way. Few of us live happily ever after. 'Even people in their forties and fifties are still expecting to find total happiness, and feeling disappointed when they don't. They have spent their lives thinking "This job will make me happy, these children will

make me happy, this relationship will make me happy..."
suddenly in mid-life they realise it isn't so.

'It's happening to the kids much earlier.

'We should be teaching young people how to cope with
disappointment, rejection, sadness and failure. Some have
learned this through family and school life. But not all of
them.'

Barry Taylor believes our society is imposing suicide on the
young as a viable solution to disappointment and despair.

'Through the media and publicity, suicide has become a
part of youth culture. Once, when kids were miserable, they
might threaten to run away. In the nineties when kids decide
nobody loves them or understands them, their conclusion is
more frequently "I want to kill myself".

'Most sixteen-year-olds know someone who has suicided. A
generation ago, nobody knew anyone young who had done
that. Today they are incredibly scared, but they accept it.
They wonder who will be next.'

Grief counsellor and psychologist Julie Dunsmore says
many young people seem to believe that nobody should have
to feel pain. 'At an age when they are wide open to
catastrophe, they don't understand how there can be
anything good about a future which may bring pain, failure
or disappointment.

'So many kids are saying they don't want to disappoint
their parents, they don't want to be disappointed again in a
relationship, they can't face being called a loser. Kids talk a
lot about their fear of being seen as losers.'

In Australia, where the youth suicide rate is the fourth
highest in the world, nobody loves a loser.

Australia and New Zealand have exceptionally high rates of
youth suicide, particularly in their rural regions. Social
analysts suggest the lack of a long, shared cultural history

and the absence of a strong sense of national confidence and identity could be a factor. It may also result from the rapid economic and social changes of these countries and their macho, do-it-yourself cultures. 'Because seeking help is seen as a weakness here,' said Barry Taylor, 'you can create all the services in the world but the people won't use them.'

God knows how hard it is for those who have lost a dearly loved young person through suicide to put this death behind them and to go on with life. God's not talking about it. But in this book, a few brave families have decided they will.

In the following pages you will read the stories of three young people, ordinary kids from ordinary families, none of them heroes, all of them loved. There are contributions from other families too – mothers and fathers who could not bear to tell all – but told enough.

Their reasons are clear and simple. They want to discourage young people from taking their lives. They want to stop the suffering and misunderstanding that is both a cause and a result of youth suicide.

They want to wipe out the stigma and explode the rumours, the secrets and the scandals that surround every one of these tragedies, so that others who have the misfortune to be touched by such awful and inexplicable death are not forced by a judgmental society to buckle even further under the weight of their already unbearable burden.

We live in a society where rampant individualism is encouraged, where goodness and morality have become old-fashioned, where family life is under incredible pressure, where the divorce rate has trebled and where a good education and the prospect of long-term employment is most likely to be restricted to the wealthy, the clever and the well-connected. We live in a country where you can't have a beaut time without booze and where it is taken for granted, even by governments, that mind-bending drugs will be used by children *(as long as they take them 'safely')*. At this time, in this place, love and good intentions are no longer enough. When it comes to equipping young people to cope with the economic, social and spiritual revolution that is propelling us through the present century and into the future, many parents feel helpless in the face of the changes which have occurred over the past thirty years.

By the time we reach the year 2000, if the current rate of death continues, another seventeen-hundred young people won't be alive to see our fabulously funded Olympic Games.

If a war was causing this sort of death rate among the flowering youth of this country the politicians, the power-mongers and the people responsible for the public purse, would be united and uncomplaining in their efforts to achieve peace.

If this many people were being killed in plane crashes, the focus of the government and the authorities would be on planning and financing sweeping measures of prevention.

If bushfires were blazing through our land, leaving this many charred bodies in their trail, billions of dollars would be spent to put out the blaze.

This is neither a war nor a holocaust. Youth suicide is an epidemic and it's happening right now, in our country regions, in our towns, in our cities, right here among us, where we can see it.

Please don't close your eyes.

COLLIN

It's not the size of the mountain but the pebble in my shoe which will limit how high I can climb.

An Indian proverb

Before the kids came along, they loved to go dancing.

Ron first saw Jan doing the Albert Hop one Saturday night down at the Palais, and he was determined to get her to teach him. 'I promised I'd show him how to do it,' she said, 'but I managed to spin it out for quite a few weeks'.

She was just under sixteen when they met; Ron did a bit of a double-take when he found out. He was nineteen, almost twenty really, and well into his apprenticeship as an electrician. Jan was straight out of school, just starting her first job with the bank. Ron thought Jan and her three sisters were pretty amazing. All that talk and laughter. It wasn't like his place, where his dad ruled the roost and he and his brother kept out of his way.

It was a bit of a culture shock but he overcame it and they danced together for three years, until Ron had the Albert Hop well under control. They were married in 1964, amid so much saving and planning and sisterly excitement that nineteen-year-old Jan may have been the only girl in Sydney to completely miss the Beatles. They built a brand new house in the neat little western Sydney suburb of Pendle Hill and when Cathy arrived, three years later, Jan gave up work to be a housewife and mother. Two years later, in 1969, their second child, Collin, was born.

JAN SCHULTZ is a tall, dignified woman of fifty-one. She has a long, well-sculpted face framed by a flipped back curtain of straight, silver-blonde hair; her voice is low and gentle and her laughter is warm but the eyes behind gold-rimmed glasses are sad. She is smart and tidy and so is her home, a comfortable blonde-brick bungalow set well back from an unsealed road in sprawling, but carefully tended, gardens. Beyond the neat row of houses are sloping hills and bushland. The beach is a few kilometres away; the city is within an hour's reach via the train or the freeway. What better place could you find to raise a family than the central coast of New South Wales?

Inside the house there is a place for everything. The couches are carefully colour-coordinated, the lamplight is soft, the carpets are fat, the bench tops gleam. Lively family photos leap along the walls, and in the living room there are scattered toys and colourful cushions. The Schultz home is highly polished and very clean but it is also cosy; the people who live within its softly-muted walls brim with affection for each other.

From the windows you can see the roses, from the kitchen comes gentle laughter, from the oven comes a crunchy aroma … it's hard to believe that any member of this family would ever want to leave.

'We were just so blessed! First a girl and then this beautiful little boy, born in twenty minutes, seven pounds two ounces – I barely made it to the hospital in time. Cathy had been a horror baby who never slept but Collin just slept, ate and sucked his thumb.

'Once he learned to walk and talk Collin was interested in everything. He followed his dad around all the time, but there was a special bond between Collin and me. He was so easy and cuddly, whereas Cathy didn't sleep properly for years and didn't much like being touched.

'He didn't like pre-school, but none of our kids did. Collin hated the puzzles and jigsaws which had fascinated Cathy, but he absolutely loved Lego and any mechanical toys.

'In 1972 we decided to take the kids and travel around Australia. Ron gave up his job and we sold our house. We bought a caravan and set off to find what life had in store for us.

'Ron had never towed a caravan before and we ran out of petrol twice before we got out of New South Wales. I wondered what I had let myself in for. He had two empty jerry cans on top of the land cruiser but he was determined to stick to his plan and this didn't include filling them until we reached the outback! We have never let him live it down.

'We went north, through Queensland and then all the way around. We went to Mount Isa, Ayers Rock, Katherine Gorge, Darwin, Fitzroy Crossing – then through South Australia. It was great. We travelled a lot at night and then we would stop in the day; Ron would get some sleep and I would play with the kids on the beach or wherever we were. Sometimes we found a base and stayed for about six weeks while Ron did a bit of electrical work.

'We all went bean picking once, but we decided that *certainly* wasn't for the Schultz family. We made about two dollars. Mind you, the kids had a ball. Ron was going around picking all the stuff the others had left behind, thinking he was doing the farmers a favour. Ron would never believe he was doing anything wrong.

'Cathy read her way around Australia, and Collin slept. He also had a lovely time, playing, fishing, crabbing, singing. We sang for hours in the car. The kids knew so many of those old songs. We had a tape of Collin and Cathy singing *The Red Red Robin*; I wish I knew where it was. I *wish* I still had it.

'We came back after about ten months because house prices were soaring and we were worried that we wouldn't have enough money to buy somewhere to live. Ron found work as an electrical contractor and we bought a really old, run-down place here on the central coast; we lived in the caravan while we did it up. It was a run-down shack really, and we intended to sell it as soon as it was ready. It was right beside a paddock and there was the bush all around. Ron and the kids outnumbered me, didn't they, so we moved in and lived there for three years. Julianne was born there in 1975.

'The children were used to a nomadic existence and the country life suited them well. There were horses about and cows – the local radio station would broadcast a message that somebody's cow was on the road and the kids would chase it home – they were very contented, very free. They went to a really nice little local school which they both loved. Well, Collin *never* really liked school but he liked being with his friends. His grades weren't good but they weren't bad either; there was nothing to tell me he wasn't coping with the work. I hit myself over the head about that now.

'We were owner-building a new house by then; Julianne was very small and then Adam was born in 1978, just after we moved in to the new place. My dad was really ill during that time – I was very busy with all this and somehow I think Collin got lost for a little while. Cathy was okay because she was so bright and such an independent, singular sort of person. But Collin slipped through the education system. Just how badly he slipped I didn't find out till years later.

'By the time Collin was seven he was entirely absorbed in mechanical things. He was always out in the yard, doing up bikes for himself and for other kids. I don't know where he got it from, as Ron hates anything to do with mechanics.

'They were wonderful years, with only a couple of ups and downs. I used to think we were like the Brady Bunch, without the divorces. Everyone thought we were a very happy family and they were right about all of us, except Collin.

'All through Collin's primary school years and in his first years of high school, Ron tried to get close to him. They would go to the gym together and then Ron started taking Collin to trampolining; he was very agile and very good at it. He had a couple of great years from ten to about thirteen – he was junior state champion and went to the national finals.

'But there was a scene when he was twelve which I've never forgotten. He was standing beside the fridge and Ron, who is quite authoritarian, was speaking to him. Collin resented whatever it was his father was saying to him. There was a huge row. I thought to myself, "This child is going to cause a lot of trouble". I was thinking of normal trouble, the kind you often expect with a boy.

'I thought the same thing on his first day at the local high school when he marched home in the middle of the day, because he had heard that another boy was going to bash him up. I asked a primary school teacher for advice and was told to get in touch with the high school to sort it out straight away. I tried. I rang the school and took him back, but the problem was never properly dealt with, and in fact continued right through Collin's high school years – mainly, I suppose, because we had taught him that it was wrong to fight.

'Collin's grades at high school were not all that bad; we didn't know how seriously behind he was until Year Nine when were called up to the school and told that he had failed to put in ten English assignments. Ten! They certainly left it for a long time before they let us know. After that it was a constant battle to get his grades up to scratch and I found myself longing for the day he left school. There was never any question of him continuing on to Year Twelve. I felt Collin's life would start when he finished with school, because he hated it there so much.

'Collin's life continued to revolve around bikes. Neighbours would knock at our door and ask if he would do up bikes for Christmas presents. "We only want to spend forty dollars," they'd say, "so tell him to do whatever he likes within that limit". He didn't get paid for the labour – he just liked doing it. He loved motorbikes of course, but he didn't have one until he built his own.

'He had a lot of friends. He was particularly popular with girls; the phone rang constantly. I couldn't believe it – we didn't do that when I was a girl. He was well-liked by the teachers who didn't have him in their classes. But none of the teachers could ever equate with Collin being Cathy's brother and he had to go all through high school in her shadow. There's no doubt that he felt it. Cathy was *very* clever.

'Collin was never in trouble for fighting or being violent and he was never rude to the teachers. He was just a clown in class, a tearaway. He wouldn't work. School was for his social life, and he had a great one. We wouldn't allow him to go out at night. Ron had rules.

'I think Collin respected us. Ron was a very authoritarian parent, although some would just call it being a responsible parent. It was the only way he knew, it was the way his father had brought him up. If I wanted to do it another way, he used to say he wouldn't be able to be a part of it. That didn't mean he was going to leave us. It just meant I'd have to bring them up without his support and I didn't think I was strong enough to do that.

'The problem was that Ron's rules were fine for kids like Cathy and Julianne and even Adam, but they didn't work with Collin. For instance, Cathy would never lie to us. She would hear Collin lying to us and she would say to him, "Why do you bother? You know they always find out the truth!" But he kept on lying.

'He lied about some of his friends, because he knew we didn't like them. He lied about where he went and what he was doing and whether parents were around at parties – that sort of thing.

'Collin was never a bad kid, never aggressive. Whatever he was feeling, he stifled it and that was the problem. I see that now. We were such a loving family, outwardly loving – we didn't call one another names, we never yelled, we never shouted – Ron and I *never* fought in front of the kids, but we rarely fought anyway. We just didn't. There was nothing to fight about. Collin must have grown up believing that you kept your good feelings out in the open and you hid your bad ones away.

'We were all openly very affectionate with each other – Ron was always grabbing me some way or another, and we'd hug in front of the children. And we'd laugh. Ron is a funny person. He *used* to be a funny person. Cath's friends thought he was a scream. But Collin's friends didn't know Ron. They never came to the house. All they knew about Ron was his rules.

'We didn't know them any better than they knew us; we were flying blind with Collin's mates.

'There was an old airstrip out in the bush near us and when he was about fifteen he wanted to go there with his friends and camp out and … drink, I suppose. I suppose that is what kids that age do. We would never allow him to go, but his friends all went and we'd watch them go past our house with their knapsacks on their backs and their tents, off for a good time.

'One night we left him to look after Julianne and Adam and when we got home *he* wasn't home, he had gone off to join his friends and he had left the little ones on their own. They were very young and he was old enough to know better, and he had been taught better. We absolutely freaked. But what do you do? How do you deal with a sixteen-year-old? How do you discipline him?

'We had an almighty row and he went out on his trampoline. I was trying to reason with him, to explain how irresponsible he had been, but he just kept bouncing up and down.

'I lost my temper. I was so angry that I threw something at him. Actually, I think it was a clock radio. It missed.

'It was a stupid thing to do. It didn't make me feel any better. I remember throwing a shoe at Ron once, which hit him, and another time I threw a carton of milk at him but I missed that time as well and it spilt all over the place, and I had to clean it up. I'm not sure if throwing three things in twenty-eight years classifies me as a thrower or not.

'We are a Christian family. Collin was confirmed into the church and he came with us until he was fourteen, but after that it became too much of a struggle to get him there.

'He left school at sixteen, after getting his school certificate and somehow passing his exams – even in English. Knowing what we know now, we still don't know how that was possible. Ron took him to lots of places and he found a temporary job at a concrete plant which enabled him to buy his first car. That's when he started getting really involved with cars. He also worked for years at McDonald's, which he hated. But Collin always had work, even if he didn't like doing it.

'When he was seventeen he fell off his pushbike and knocked three teeth out. He had beautiful teeth, and it cost more than $3000 to repair them with crowns. It was a taste of what was to come.

'He didn't smoke at all. He hated smoking; his grandfather (Ron's dad) smoked all the time and died of lung cancer. I don't think Collin ever smoked and don't believe he started drinking until he was about twenty. He hated the club life, which makes up a big part of the social scene around here.

'Then he got an apprenticeship to be a fitter-mechanic. I cried when he rang to tell me. It could not have been better for Collin if he had won Lotto. At last he had achieved something that he really wanted.

'He didn't get it through the normal channels. A friend of ours persuaded the company in question to interview Collin, even though he wasn't doing the required course at the technical college. The company fellow wasn't keen at all until he talked to Collin, who arrived on the motorbike he had built himself from scratch, armed with photographs of all the mechanical projects he had completed. Collin's experience put him head and shoulders above all the other applicants, so he got the job. He was also a lovely kid, with a big, friendly smile and people liked him and wanted to help him.

'Of course getting the apprenticeship meant he had to go to tech and, like school, that was his downfall. To get through any kind of course you have to be able to read.'

RON SCHULTZ is trim and taut, a compact man with thinning silver hair, a tanned face and a polite blue-eyed grin which is sometimes too painfully bright. He is a disciplined person who works hard; no job is too small to be done well. His garden is immaculate, stray blades of grass flinch as he hurries up the front path. He has equipped the garden shed as a small gymnasium in order to keep fit and he runs every morning. His father was a German labourer who had little to do with his two sons, and spent his weekends over bets and beers. His mum sometimes came to see them play sport at school, but not often. They didn't have a car.

Until he met Jan, Ron thought he would spend his life as a confirmed bachelor. He was over-awed by her household of women and it was a relief to take her away from them and to set themselves up as an independent family. When their pigeon-pair of babies arrived, he could barely believe his good fortune.

Ron gave up smoking when Collin was born. He gave up drinking a few years later, when the children reached an impressionable age. He was determined to be a better father than his own.

'I was always very black-and-white with the kids. I didn't praise them enough, I realise that now. Of the two older ones, one excelled and one didn't. It was as simple as that. Then we had the same pattern with the younger two. I never made a fuss about it.

'When they did something wrong I would warn them. If they didn't stop by the time I had counted to three they would get a smack. I rarely had to smack them, but when I did I smacked them hard. I believed that was the way you brought up kids to do as they were told.

'When he was fifteen I clipped Collin over the ears for doing something wrong. Afterwards I said to myself, "Ron, you're wrong. You're not teaching your kids to stand up for themselves". I went to Collin's room and apologised. I said, "I'm sorry. You are too old to be smacked now. In future I will ask you not to do things but it will be up to you whether you obey me. I will never hit you again".

'We did lots of things together. I took him to trampolining three times a week. When he was sixteen I took him to New Zealand and we had a ball.

'I was pretty hard on him, but you want your kids to do well, you want to give them a good start in life and you want them to do better than you.

'As he grew older, Collin started putting up barriers between him and me. We could have a perfectly reasonable conversation about why he shouldn't do something and two days later he'd be doing it again. Why? "Because I want to." He had a short attention span.

'I honestly believe he started doing up bikes because he knew I was no good at it; he knew I couldn't stand over his shoulder telling him what he should do, correcting his mistakes. He was a very determined boy; he had plenty of grit. We refused to let him buy a motorbike so he decided to build one himself. I passed him on the way home one afternoon, struggling along on his pushbike, carrying a motorbike frame on his shoulders. That's how he started.

'Collin was still riding a pushbike when he was harassed by the police for riding on the wrong side of the road. He came home petrified, trembling and shaking and crying. They had run him off the road and they contacted us and told us we had to take him to the station. I suppose they were only trying to scare him into riding safely, but that started him off. He hated the police from then on.'

Since she was ten years old, CATHY SCHULTZ has been an uncannily perceptive and intuitive young woman. Now twenty-nine, she is smaller than her siblings, pale skinned, brown haired; she has never been very interested in her own appearance or that of anyone else. Her mother believes she sees people only from the inside.

Life has not been kind to Cathy, yet now and then an irrepressible sense of humour bubbles through and her thoughtful monologue is interrupted with a deep, husky chuckle. It's a good sound in this house.

'We had a great time when we were kids. There was the trip around Australia – then coming back and settling up here, with the fields all round and a family living right next door so we had ready-made friends straight away.

'We used to go on long walks at night after dinner. Sometimes we took our scooters. When we were older Collin and I used to get up at six a.m. and run with Dad. We did it for a couple of years until we ran out of steam.

'One Christmas when we were very small we crept into the lounge room to see our presents and there was a bike for

Collin. He was beside himself with excitement; he wanted to ride it straight away, but it was still pitch-black outside. He nearly went crazy, sitting there amid wall-to-wall presents, while we gorged ourselves on lollies and waited for the sun to come up so he could get on that bike.

'Collin wasn't naughty but he was a daredevil. He was dared to eat the inside of a swamp lily once and he came home screaming, thinking he was going to die because it had been all peppery – he did some stupid things.

'He wasn't a fighter. Collin always assumed he would get beaten up if he fought. I remember Dad trying to teach him to fight so he would stand up for himself. Once he left school he got into the body building – he had shoulders out to here – so nobody picked on him much after that.

'We fought very rarely, but when we did it was to the death. We didn't do it when Mum was around. He threw a typewriter at me once. Another time he attacked me with a slide screen. Our friends couldn't believe two such quiet kids could turn so feral. But we were a bit scared of ourselves so we stopped fighting. We were both afraid of what happened when we crossed that line.

'We loved each other but Collin and I had nothing in common. From the age of about fourteen he decided it was an embarrassment to have a family at all. You know – four paces behind the rest of us at the shops. And there were always all these girls hanging around him so he couldn't be seen with us.

'He was different with Julianne and Adam because he doted on them. I remember Adam once falling off this retaining wall and Collin racing to get Dad and screaming and screaming at him to hurry. Dad is always so low key, so calm, he has enormous self-control. He refuses to fight because when he breaks, he really breaks. But Collin used to panic about things; he couldn't keep the lid on his feelings, he was too volatile. A lot of the time when he was older he had so much rage and frustration in him, he couldn't control it.'

Tall, vivacious, dark and pretty, JULIANNE WAIT loves being married. Just twenty years old and a student at the University of Newcastle, her parents raised few objections when she told them she wanted to marry Robbie Wait, whom she had met when she was in Year Eleven at school. Jan and Ron feel they no longer have the right to refuse their children any chance at happiness.

Julianne is studying to be a teacher of children with special needs. In particular, she is going to teach them to read.

'We had a big dirt room under our other house and when I was little I would go down there and watch Collin working on the bikes. He let me help him; I'd scratch around in the dirt for old nuts and bolts ... I don't suppose he ever used them.

'Collin was so cool. He was a rebel without a cause. Girls would make friends with me just so that they could meet him. He was *so* good looking. He was in sixth class when I was in kindergarten – he and his mates would protect me. He was a good big brother.

'Our parents were very strict. They had rules. A lot of our friends, their parents don't have rules and they can do what they want. Our parents weren't like that. Collin got into a lot of trouble so they had to come down hard on him.

'He wasn't introverted but he didn't say a lot; he was cool, he didn't have to say much. Collin just *was*. By the time I got to high school he had left but he had this incredible reputation; all the teachers wanted to know if I was going to be like Collin or like Cathy. In fact I was somewhere in the middle.

'I think Collin's troubles started at school. His problems were not picked up. I know now that there are ways he could have been helped. He was always making comments about not being able to write properly, about being dumb. But nobody realised how bad it was. He was so good at other things.

'I had a very happy childhood; I always felt loved and secure. As far as I knew, Collin's was the same. He had everything – he could do anything with bikes and cars, he had beautiful girlfriends and he was so popular. Even after he left school, the senior girls knew about him. They let me sit on the back seat of the bus, so they could get to know more about him. It was my ambition to be as cool and as popular as Collin.'

When Collin heard Jaakko's name read out in the second year of high school, he assumed the new boy would be foreign and black. He was half right. JAAKKO and his family had come to Australia from Finland; he was short and fair and desperate for his growth spurt.

It came. Jaakko is now six feet tall, a sandy haired, good looking man of twenty-seven, with the broad shoulders and narrow waist of a carpenter who works hard at his trade. Together the two young revheads used to make quite an impression on the local female population, but the boys took for granted the pleasures offered by feminine flesh. They were much more obsessed with the mechanics of speed.

'Collin and I used to get booted out of science class together at high school; it was never anything major and more my fault than his. Making silly noises mainly. We used to wag school towards the end of the year and go swimming at the railway dam. I was okay at the schoolwork for a while, but there were so many kids there who were out of control it was hard to learn. The teachers would always be going off – it was a pretty wild class. I fell down in maths but I had a good imagination so I was pretty good at English. I don't know if Collin had any trouble with the work. He didn't talk about it.

'It was more important to decide what you were going to do in the afternoons and weekends. We were really interested in BMX bikes first, then we went on to motorcross bikes and then to motorbikes. Collin bought a mangled mess of a bike off somebody and he worked on it for hours and got it going.

'Collin was pretty popular with the girls; he always had women chasing him. He only went with the best looking ones. I was a late bloomer; I was shorter than a lot of the other fellas in high school and I was shy, I'd get the shakes – at first I couldn't even look at girls without going to pieces. I got a few after a while but never as many as Collin.

'I'm the youngest of six and my parents were pretty old-fashioned; I was kept at home a lot when I was younger. Collin had been out and about a lot more than me. I met Lindy when I was sixteen and we've been together ever since.

'We used to all meet up at the old airstrip a lot, to watch guys rally their cars. We'd ride our bikes up there and we went on some long rides together. Collin got booked for speeding on his road bike.

'At the beginning of Year Ten I left school and went to be a labourer; then I went to tech. I wanted to be a mechanic but I couldn't get into the course, so I've ended up as a form-work carpenter.

'Collin left school at the end of that year; we spent more time together once we started working on our cars. Collin was a cheerful person. He would snap pretty quickly when something went wrong but he got over things fast. We used to hassle each other all the time.

'Collin loved to speed. When you've just got your licence and you've spent months hotting up a car all you want to do is drive it fast. You don't do it in town. You go out on the highway or out into the country where it's quiet. Collin was no worse than the rest of us. We were all ratbags, the whole lot of us.'

JASON

Let none tell me the past is wholly gone.
Now is so small a part of time, so small a part
Of all the race years that have moulded me.

From *The Past* by Oodgeroo of the tribe Noonuccal
(formerly known as Kath Walker)

It's Saturday morning at the Connors' white-painted brick house in Martini Street and there's a lot going on.

Out the back, where vegetables and flowers, bike bits and junked toys sprout in hectic profusion, the dogs are barking, mad with excitement at the prospect of a walk with Erin – satin-black hair, dungarees, a friendly smile – and her plump and pony-tailed girlfriend. Charmaine's new baby, Huntar (named after someone gorgeous in 'The Bold and the Beautiful') is gurgling in her pram, which is competing with Peter's crutches as the biggest obstacle in the crowded hallway. The cricket moans from the television in the dim lounge room, where the father of the house is struggling to get up from the lumpy couch without putting any weight on his injured foot. Kurt – tall and lean, flame-haired – is in the kitchen, making himself a sandwich, home unexpectedly after ten days of work with the drilling rig because there's some sort of strike. The kettle's whooping for Ceane, who is expected to drop in soon and Stacey is due home any minute too, because it's a big night for the social club and she needs time to get all dressed up like a sore toe. Ashleigh – slight, fair, ten years old – bursts into the big bright dining room at the back of the house, wanting money for lollies if she has to go to the shop.

Keiran – skinny, lively, and the youngest at eight (if you don't count Huntar, and Ceane's little Jessica) – is hanging around. He can't tear his gaze from the big photograph that is lying on the long dining table. It's a picture of Jason, his eldest brother; Jason, his hero – an olive-skinned boy with a shy, sweet smile and kind eyes, averted in embarrassment before the unseen camera.

A few tiny, undistinguished photos of the Connor kids when they were all small, stand in frames in the lounge room, but Keiran hasn't noticed them much. It's the first time for months that anyone has brought out this nice big picture of his brother. There are some school photos on the table as well and Keiran examines them curiously. Straight rows of boys in ties and Jason, not much older than Keiran is now, rounder than the rest of the class, and chubby, with curly black hair. Keiran is not familiar with any of this. Ties. Straight lines. His wraith-thin big brother covered in cushions of flesh. None of these pictures are part of his world any more.

Presiding over the noise, the mess, the sandwich making, the kettle, the crying, the questions and the obstacle course – 'Someone push open the back door so Charmaine can get the pram out there into the fresh air!' – is Lee Connor*, forty-three, wife of Peter and mother of nine children, six of whom still live at home. Calm, good-humoured, casual but firm each time a decision is demanded, Lee sits smoking cigarettes and drinking tea at her big table, alternately dispensing advice, instructions, laughter, discipline, chocolate bars and conversation.

A solid and handsome woman, sallow-skinned with short, thick black hair, Lee grew up in this place. She and Peter have raised eight children here. Everyone knows them. Young local people speak almost enviously of the Connor family – and then fall silent in confusion, wondering how they can still feel this way. 'Mr and Mrs Connor always had these rules, so you knew exactly how far you could push', 'Their mum once let us kids put up a tent in her lounge room and sleep there overnight', 'I loved going there to play. There was always lots of love around'.

The town is surrounded by mountains. Immense, still, majestic, their spires appear soft and smoky blue at the rim of the distant city but nothing is as it seems down there. Up close the mountains are black and red and rough, craggy and crusted with olive-green bush. They are omnipresent. The mines gave this town its character; the mountains provide its soul.

LEE CONNOR was taken from her Aboriginal mother when she was three years old and transported into these mountains by train. All she remembers is that a kind priest gave her some books to read on the journey – and that it was so freezing when she arrived she thought she might die from the cold.

She was put in the care of a white family with three sons. 'Everyone in the town thought what a lucky little girl I was,' said Lee, 'being taken in and treated so kindly by a "proper" family'.

In fact her new 'mother' *was* relatively kind to her and the boys, who were much older, left her alone. She slept in the same bed as the woman and her husband but the man came to bed much earlier than his wife and Lee clearly remembers being sexually abused by him when she was very young. He died within a year of her arrival and Lee, the daughter her foster mother had never had, became the main focus of the woman's life.

She met her real mother again at the age of eleven and was permitted to go with her into the country for a holiday. Here Lee saw her black grandmother for the first time.

'I had never seen a black person in my life,' she said. 'When I spoke to my grandmother I suddenly became aware that I had a real identity of my own. I had been a withdrawn and unhappy child. When I found my grandmother I also found myself.

'At the same time, I realised I had lost my culture. Because even though I discovered who I was, I was uncomfortable with my real family. They were different from me – just too different.'

Lee wanted to come back to her home in the mountains. Her life there, her friends, her school, even her other 'mother', were more familiar to her than the life she experienced in the outback town.

But things were never the same with her foster mother again.

At the age of fourteen, while walking home through a park after visiting a girlfriend, Lee was attacked, threatened with a knife and raped. Nobody saw. Nobody told. It took her until 3 a.m. to stagger home. She put herself to bed. She said she didn't want to get beaten.

A few weeks later, when she discovered she was pregnant, the story had to come out. Her foster mother tried hot baths and gin to bring on an abortion but her efforts failed. She told Lee she was a slut, which the girl could not understand. She had not, after all, been raped by choice.

Lee was not allowed to return to high school, so her education ceased halfway through Year Seven. Her foster mother made arrangements for the baby to be adopted, but when her son was born, Lee persuaded the hospital authorities to allow her to contact her real mother, who arrived in the town a week later, offering to take her grandson and bring him up as her own.

Lee had not been permitted to see or touch her baby. When her mother took him home from the hospital she was allowed to hold him in her arms for the first and last time. She would not see him again for many years and when they eventually met again, he was more like a younger brother than a son.

Ashamed and too embarrassed to send Lee back to school, her foster mother found her a job in a factory and covered the young woman's shapely body with childish frocks, insisting on white socks and buckled shoes, in an effort to restore some semblance of white respectability to her life.

Four years later, after what she describes as a one night stand, Lee again became pregnant, this time by choice. At seventeen, still grieving for the son she had lost, she was determined to have a baby of her own, one she could love and keep. Her second son was born in October, 1970. She called him Jason.

'When I decided I wanted a baby I didn't see any reason to have a father around. I knew I could give him all the love he needed.

'At first my foster mother wouldn't let me come home with him. She had expected me to have the baby adopted. I stayed with a friend for a couple of weeks but then she asked me to come back to her. She was a strange woman. She is dead now but even with the wisdom of hindsight I can't understand the way she thought.

'She loved Jason and he loved her. She looked after him so I could go back to work.

'Jason was still only a baby when Peter came to board with the people who lived next door. We became good friends, although I was never allowed to go out anywhere and I was still wearing shoes and socks and not being allowed to wear make-up or anything – at eighteen. Peter treated Jason wonderfully, even though he had never had anything to do with children before.

'My foster mother hated Peter. She said he was a red-headed bastard who only wanted to do – you know – *that*. She was very old-fashioned. To get out of the place and away from her I went to live with Peter. Ceane was born two years later. When she was six weeks old, Peter and I were married.

'I knew from the first time I met Peter that he was for me, for the rest of my life. Peter felt the same way and he accepted Jason as his child and never treated him any differently to the others. He changed his nappies, he fed him bottles, he looked after him when we went out.

'Peter was with the railways and we travelled around a lot when the older children were very small – six weeks here, three months there. Jason had started school by then, so he stayed in town with my foster mother – his nanna he called her. We came home every second weekend to see him. This went on for about eighteen months.

'At school, he got there but he struggled. He was the class clown. He had a bit of a weight problem when he was eight or nine and I think it must have affected his self-esteem, although at the time you would never have guessed it. He was quite dark as well, but he never told me if he was teased about that as well.

'As Jason grew older, Peter took him to soccer, and hockey. This is a very sporty town. Jason, Ceane, Charmaine and Stacey played sport every weekend and we would all go and watch. I always had a baby who had to be dragged out into the cold – so after a while Peter just went on his own. Then, when we got to Kurt we stopped the kids doing Saturday sport. They still did it at school but weekends were getting too hectic.

'After Ceane and Charmaine we had Stacey, Kurt and Erin. Ashleigh arrived five years after that and Keiran, the youngest, was born two years later.

'No, we're not Catholics. I had planned to stop at four but I suppose I just wanted the big, loving family that I had missed out on as a child. Peter didn't want this many kids, of course he didn't, but he is a very cooperative, loving sort of person and to make me happy I think he just thought, "Oh well, what's another one?" We did send the kids to Catholic high schools. In fact the younger ones have gone to Catholic schools all the way through.

'I used to do bar work at night, when Peter was at home to look after the kids. It helped a bit for me to work part-time – we had a lot of mouths to feed. Nobody apart from us ever looked after our children. We didn't go out much but it didn't bother us. One of us has always been at home for the kids. Not knowing how a normal family operates, I just thought that was the only way to do it.

'When I was twenty-six I started having counselling because of all the stuff that had happened to me. I asked the counsellor when I should tell Jason where he had come from and he said just before puberty was a good time. So when he was eleven years old I told Jason that Peter wasn't his real father. He was very upset. He cried so much. I told him I loved him and how much I had wanted him, but he still cried.

'I thought he was ready, but he just broke his heart about it. Peter was really upset with me, too. He couldn't see any reason why Jason had to know he wasn't his real father. He told Jason he loved him dearly.

'I just thought this was a small town and he would be better off finding out from his mother than from someone else. As it was, his nanna told him a week later in a not very nice way. So I was glad I had done it first.

'Eventually I told him the whole story. Jason never wanted to find his real father or anything. He said Peter was his dad and that was that.

'He knew about his Aboriginality. They all knew about that.

'He was plump and jolly and he clowned his way through high school. He loved bikes and because we didn't have much money he would go out and wash windows and offer to wash cars to earn enough to get what he wanted. He was very tidy and clean. I suppose he got that from me. I was used to scrubbing floors for hours on my knees and then going back and polishing the lot until it glowed. Jason wasn't afraid of hard work either.

'But because he was the eldest I suppose I took advantage of him. He was mentally mature, and he was gentle and cheerful. Jason was the one I could ask to look after the babies while I was cooking tea. He was very responsible and Peter was often away on shift work – but he often offered to help. He didn't complain.

'The kids all looked up to Jason. He gave them advice behind our backs. He made the kids laugh. He joked with them and tickled them, he had a lot to do with them. Even when he grew up and left home, he was so close to the rest of them. No matter how broke he was, he always had presents for them under the Christmas tree.

'With hindsight, I think he probably did have problems at school, but he kept them to himself. He was teased a lot about his weight, I think. That was the only thing about Jason that ever seriously worried me. But he was always so jovial.

'I remember when he was sixteen we had one big blue. He put his fists up and he said to me, "Mum, I feel like hitting you". Then he looked really frightened and ran away. He came back a long time later and told me he loved me and he was sorry.

'I wouldn't let him leave school unless he had a full-time job. I didn't want him to get into the dole routine. He went to Telecom as a linesman and he worked very hard. He was there for about five years and in that time he bought two cars. He was very independent, but he got into debt. Then again, all kids get into debt when they first start getting a pay cheque – it wasn't serious.

'Once he started work he became addicted to junk food.

Because of his hours, he was no longer coming home to a hot meal on the table every night – so he bought pies and hamburgers and Coke. I told him to come home for a meal before he went out to enjoy himself – it would have been cheaper for him.

'Jason went around with a mixed crowd, although as far as I know, he never had a girlfriend. He was shy with girls but very respectful of women in general. He was always very concerned about people who were down and out. When a girlfriend of one of his mates had a baby, he went to see her every day in the hospital.

'He was a happy person. He always had a smile for everyone. But he was a straight talker. He was never afraid to stick up for himself.

'At seventeen he moved into a house with some friends, but he would come and see us regularly.

'Jason obviously had more serious self-esteem problems than anyone realised, especially when it came to his weight and possibly when it came to his Aboriginality. People gave him a hard time about being eligible for Abstudy and things, not that he ever applied for anything. Ceane was always very proud of being an Aboriginal; I think Jason respected it underneath. One day a year he took a holiday on National Aborigines Day.

'When it came to being an individual, living on his own, trying to get what he really wanted out of life, working really hard, it just didn't come as easily as he had expected.

'When Keiran was about seventeen months old I found out I had breast cancer. I had a mastectomy and I was in hospital for quite a while. The kids would come to see me but Jason only visited once and wouldn't come again. I think it upset him more than he let on.

'He was still very close to his nanna and to her invalid son, Fred*, who had been like an uncle to Jason. When my foster mother became ill and disabled, he actually moved down there to look after Nanna and Fred, to take the pressure off me. I was studying at the time. When Keiran was old enough I had enrolled for a three year social science course at a TAFE college. But I was going to my foster mother's house to look after her and her son; I had to shower and bath them and all that and it was hard work, so Jason helped me out. He was very caring. Eventually we had to put them both in a home. My foster mother died a year later and Fred had a heart attack and died twelve months after that. Jason missed them very much.

'When he was twenty-three he changed jobs and went to work as a linesman with the State Rail Authority. That's when he moved into a house of his own, in Bracken *, a little town a few miles up the mountain.

'I thought he was starting to eat better because he started losing weight and whenever I went up there, I'd see fruit lying around and meat out thawing for tea. He started to look really really good.

'It wasn't until a couple of weeks before the crisis came that I realised Jason was seriously miserable. I was back in the workforce myself by then; I was doing welfare work with women in crisis. On that particular day I was working up in the mountains, not far from where he was based. He came to see me. He told me he had been to the doctor's and the doctor had told him he was depressed and was considering prescribing antidepressants. Jason had taken medication for depressants before, but he said they didn't work.

'By then he had lost so much darn weight it was unbelievable. He was like a bloody ... well, he didn't look good any more, that's for sure. What he did was wear bulky clothes. Really bulky clothes, so you couldn't tell what he looked like underneath them. I thought he was going through a bad time because all his friends were getting married or in relationships and there were kids coming along for them. I thought he might be thinking, "Oh shit all my friends are married and here I am, a bachelor, living in a pad by myself".

'I was a bit surprised when he asked me to lend him fifty dollars so he could buy some lunch, some petrol and drive down to the town to pick up a cheque from the bank. He had arranged a loan from the bank to pay off all his debts. It wasn't that he was behind in his rent or any of his repayments – he just wanted to pay them all off so he only had to worry about one loan and that would cover his car insurance and his rego and everything as well.

'I thought if he was worried about his bills and all I had to do was lend him fifty dollars so he could clear them all up, everything would be fine.

'But he said something really strange to me that day. We were having this talk in a women's refuge, where I was working, and he said, "Mum, is it really that bad for these women? Do they really have to leave their families and their homes?" It wasn't like him to be so serious.

'But really, at no time did I ever really worry about Jason. I mean, my work involves talking to people who regularly attempt suicide. And I never once considered that Jason had that in mind.

'Another thing that threw me off was the conversation I had with a friend of Jason's whose grandfather committed suicide. She told me what a comfort Jason had been to her. He told her he couldn't understand why anybody would kill themselves. "You'd have to be on your last legs to do a thing like that", he said to her.'

It's Saturday afternoon at the Connors' and there's a lot going on.

A communal howl of horror follows Stacey down the hall because her long, long legs are burnt bright pink and how will she hide them at the club tonight? With a bang, a crash and a lot of wallops, Erin and her girlfriend come back with the dogs, having walked all through town and up into the bush for more than two hours.

'Can Peta stay over? Can we camp out? Can we put up the tent in the yard? Please Mum? Please Dad?' Fifteen and full of energy, there is no sign of the recalcitrant teenager about Erin. 'I'd love to be a writer. What's it like to be a writer? I'm good at English.'

Does she want to tell us about Jason? 'I'm not really one for talking about it. It's just something that happened. Mum, is there anything to eat?'

PETER CONNOR makes no comment on Erin's answer. He sits and listens. He is big and bulky, observant, considerate and more quietly concerned with what is going on in this crowded house than his bristling eyebrows and macho moustache suggest. He knows where everybody is and when they are due home, where the baking dishes are kept, how much sleep the baby has had and, astonishingly, where Stacey's can of hairspray is hiding. He washes up formidable loads of dishes without complaint. He explains modestly that he's a bit more in touch than usual at the moment because he's been off work with a broken foot. A transformer fell on it at the mines.

He pulls up a chair at the table and chuckles at the sight of Erin and her friend Peta, out in the yard, dancing with the dogs. His eyes are dark and gentle as he slips into memories of other Saturdays.

'Ceane used to give Jason hell. She used to stir him up something fierce. He was chasing her one weekend and she slammed the front door on him and he smashed his hand right through the glass.

'Generally though, he was harmless and happy-go-lucky. He took a lot of rubbish from his siblings; he was pretty placid. He got on specially well with Stacey. She was the youngest for a long time and he was seven years older; they had a special bond.

'We used to live up in North Street, right under the mountain. All the local kids would go camping up there, they'd light fires in the caves and barbecue their sausages. You could see the flames for miles – half the time we were worried they'd set fire to the whole bloody mountain.

'Jason used to ride his trail bike up there. He knew everybody and they knew him; that's what happens when you've been in a place as long as we've been here and you have this many kids.

'We took them all on holidays every year. Jason was a real beach person. He loved the surf. When you live on top of a mountain and you suddenly see all this lovely water – there was no holding him back. Lee would sit on the beach, terrified that he was going to drown. Even when the older ones left home they came on holidays with us when they could.

'When Ceane was a teenager we found out she was involved with drugs and we focused all our attention on her. We put so much energy into trying to solve her problems, but we assumed the rest were okay. Maybe Jason's troubles began to develop then and we didn't notice because we were so worried about Ceane.

'He wasn't a drinker. The only time Jason drank alcohol instead of Coke was the night before his twenty-first birthday. Some mates gave him a bottle of ouzo and he had that. It didn't go down too well and the next night, when we had a bit of a party up at the hotel, he only drank orange juice. We had a karaoke machine and everything. We all had a great night; it was a good party.

'It wasn't long after that he started losing weight.

'He used to carry a calorie counter book in his pocket. He could tell you how many calories were in any food he saw you eat – even just a biscuit. He'd come around and have a cup of coffee with you and he'd tell you how many calories were in the Tim Tam you offered him.

'Why he couldn't sleep I don't know but he saw a few doctors about that. They told him he was depressed and gave him pills. They never told him you had to stay on them for the long term if you wanted them to do any good. He'd get a boost from the pills and then he would decide he didn't need them any more and down he would go again.

'He was a social smoker. It only dawned on us slowly that he was smoking marijuana too – he'd probably been smoking pot for about three years. The last doctor that he saw told him he couldn't give him antidepressant tablets unless his system was clear of marijuana. So he gave it up and he had a blood test a few weeks later which showed he didn't have any drugs left in him.

'By this time he looked bloody terrible. But he was really cunning about the way he dressed. You couldn't pick up what he looked like under his clothes. He would come around to see us at dinner time. There's always extra food available in a big family like this. You'd say, "Grab a knife and fork and have dinner with us", but he'd say he was going to eat with his mates. Later we found out he'd say to his mates that he couldn't eat with them because he was coming round to eat with us.

'He must have been so hungry, but it obviously wasn't food that Jason needed.'

MAZ

There was a little girl and she had a little curl
Right in the middle of her forehead.
When she was good she was very very good
But when she was bad she was horrid.

A nursery rhyme

'One night when she was young and she couldn't stand living at home any more, our mother threw a huge plate of spaghetti bolognaise at her father. It hit him full in the face and when the plate fell down and twirled around on the table, he was wearing mince and tomatoes and there were ropes of spaghetti hanging over his big hooked nose.

Mum then stood up, said goodbye politely to her browbeaten mother and her two spoilt brothers and ran away with the bloke who eventually became our father.

Me and Edward and Jilly have heard this story so often we all feel as if we were there. The moral is supposed to be that everyone is allowed to do one bad thing in their life, so it was okay for her to throw her dinner at her old man. In actual fact, chucking the spag bol wasn't nearly as bad and as stupid as marrying our father and giving birth to us three kids and, as a result, lumbering herself for life with a whole heap of bad things, but nobody ever mentions *that*. It would be the truth, and we're all really good at avoiding the truth in our family.

Diana has told me to keep a diary, only I'm not to show it to anybody, not even her. Diana's the school counsellor. This is supposed to get out all my bad feelings in a safe way.

She says it will work for me because I've always done so well at school. Kids like me are not supposed to get top marks – I am the exception to the general rule. Of course I don't work as hard as Edward or Jilly but you know, I'm not a total spaz.

This is actually a pretty crumby looking exercise book, so there's no way I'm writing Dear Diary or Dear Anything for that matter, so I'll just keep going.

Our father is a con-man and a drunk and a liar and a womaniser. Other than that he is a thoroughly lovable chap, tall, dark and very handsome, with black bouffy hair and big sexy eyes and lovely clothes. He always smells delicious. He always smells much better than me. Our mother used to be very pretty until she got thin and worried looking; she had the most beautiful crinkly smile, like that lady on 'Playschool', and dark brown curly hair. In photos of them when they were young I always thought they looked more like brother and sister than husband and wife.

I've only ever lived in a house once and that was on a holiday. We moved around a lot when we were kids and we always lived in flats or units. Our father changed jobs fairly frequently, according to how quickly the various companies he sold things for found out he was cheating them or feeling up their female staff. What Dad was best at selling was himself.

Our mother worked from when Jilly started school; before that she was always paranoid about us all ending up out on the street without a bean to scratch ourselves with (why would you scratch yourself with a bean, or have I got that mixed up with something else?) so as soon as she had her youngest child off her hands she went off to her Morbid Job. Of course she had to change jobs every time we moved but she always called her work her Morbid Job, so that we were never in any doubt that by going off and leaving us with babysitters like dreadful Mrs Kemp, our nosy neighbour with BO, she was actually making a huge sacrifice for us. The main thing here was that we shouldn't make her feel guilty. She was Doing the Right Thing. It was For Our Own Good. That was that. We all hated Kreepy Kempy. She stank and she smoked and she drank Mum's sherry. It was much better when Edward was considered old enough to be a latch key babysitter.

Edward was always the responsible one. The brain. The nerd. Head always in a book. Beanpole, glasses, sprouty hair – you know the type. You'd like to hate him but he was too nice, too harmless. Anyway, he probably wouldn't have noticed. He hardly ever noticed anything. He was always in his room reading and when they got him a computer he was always into that, staring at the screen. He never looked you in the eye. Now I'm older I've worked it out. Edward perfected the art of ignoring everything that went on around him, because that was easier than noticing what was happening.

I am four years younger than Edward and not at all like him. I'm little and chunky and they say I have my mother's crinkly eyes; before I shaved my head my hair used to be thick and straight, not like my parents' or Edward's. The fact that I don't look like anyone wasn't so noticeable until Jilly came along and turned out to be a female clone of Edward. I was pretty sure from an early age that I must have been adopted. There were Mum and Dad looking like twins and Edward and Jilly looking like a second set, thin and pale and intelligent. And then me. The fat little cushion in the middle.

I wasn't only different to look at. The big problem they had with me from a very early age was that I did my one bad thing when I was about two, which was crapping in my cot and then crawling out and painting the walls with it, and then I did a lot more bad things, which wasn't how it was meant to be. It didn't fit in with our mother's rules about the general scheme of things.

Edward had all these bears – don't laugh – when he was young, and he looked after them so carefully. Jilly had dolls and she was the same with them. She washed them and combed them; she kept their clothes in labelled plastic bags, for shit's sake. I had one fat doll, called Elizabeth, after the Queen. Mum named her. Mum named all our dolls. I actually called her Bimbo. We were living in a first floor flat at the time and my favourite game was throwing Bimbo Elizabeth out of the window, and racing down the stairs to see if I could catch her before she landed. I never did. Her eyes fell out the first time I tried it and she had this blank stare. When I got sick I used to dream about Bimbo Elizabeth's stare all the time. But I kept chucking her out the window. Jilly hated it. Sometimes she even cried, and tried to comfort the doll. That's the sort of fruitcake I have for a sister.

I used to run away a lot when I was little, but never very far. I mainly went when Mum and Dad were in the middle of a row, because they never noticed anything then, nor heard anything neither, with all the shouting and screaming that went on. Edward used to shut his door – he always got a room to himself because he was the boy. When she was old enough to understand what was going on, Jilly would go in the shower and sing really loudly. She had a terrible voice. I didn't think running away was any worse than what they did, but it seemed to worry Mum more when she found out and – what was worse – Other People sometimes had to be told I was missing. Having Other People know anything at all was wrong with our family was our mother's worst nightmare. The other complication was that when I went, I often didn't wear any clothes. You can do that in Brisbane, which is where we lived then, because it's warm for a lot of the year.

I think I was quite a happy little kid, actually, and I always had heaps of friends. I always liked looking after people so when they had problems I would bring them home and try to cheer them up. I hated injustice. I remember this girl coming to school with a handknitted Broncos beanie on her head; it was identical to Dougie Robbins' beanie and I took her down behind the toilets and I shook her and shook her because I thought she had pinched it. Anyway, it turned out she hadn't. Her mother had knitted it for her. I felt like a nit but I was glad, too, because this girl's mother didn't look the type to do anything for her. Our mother did things for us all the time – sewed school costumes, knitted jumpers, ironed everything, cooked huge fattening meals which had no effect on Edward or Jilly but turned me into Porky Pig. Our father was hardly ever home at night, so I suppose she just liked to keep busy so she wouldn't get lonely.

We weren't supposed to bring people home after school but once Edward was in charge you could do anything. He never noticed. Everyone liked coming to our place. Our parents never stayed in one place long enough to save much money but my mother had very good taste and our flats were very nicely furnished with everything cheap but matching. We were the same. Edward and Jilly and I were always neatly dressed, we always matched or else we were colour-coordinated. It all went with the image that we were a Nice Family. The best thing anyone could say to our mother was that her children always looked *smart*. She cared more about us looking smart than being smart.

I liked school. I enjoyed learning. I listened a lot and even with changing schools a fair bit, I was almost always near the top of the class. I have – well, I used to have – a really good memory for facts and garbage and that. I haven't been so good at remembering stuff lately.

Our mother had all these special routines which went with being a Nice Family. For instance, when we lived in Melbourne, every Sunday we went to our uncle and auntie's for tea. You can't imagine how we kids hated those long drives to the relatives' place. Our mother and father never spoke to each other, they never had a conversation. It was such a relief to get there, so Mum could talk to her sister-in-law and Dad could talk to our uncle and everybody pretended everything was cool.

It was worse when we went on holidays. They were the worst time for rows. Our parents couldn't be together for long without fighting. The long drives to and from the coast were awful. I hated them. All that silence, or if a row started, it would last the whole way.

One year, I will never forget, we were driving home from a week at the beach and it hadn't been too bad. It was late in the afternoon and we were cruising along this straight country road and all the clouds were pink. Dad started to sing. He had a very good voice and he used to sing quite a bit in the shower. Suddenly Mum started to sing with him. Our mother never sang. As soon as she started I could see who Jilly had inherited her voice from. It was that Beatles song, *Norwegian Wood*. They sang it together, all of it, and he harmonised and everything. I sat in the back with my mouth open. I was just gobsmacked. I looked at Jilly, but she was asleep. Then I saw Edward. He had his head in a book, as usual. But his face was bright red. He just sat there, with his eyes riveted to the page and his face the colour of the sunset.

When they finished nobody said a word. We just kept driving.

After Brisbane we moved to Adelaide, which was horrible, but I soon made some friends and it was okay. Six months later we moved again. All my friends? Gone. Bang. This time we went to Melbourne. Mum got a job again but the suburb where we lived was a long way out of the city. She missed her Brisbane friends a lot. I remember very clearly one Saturday afternoon when I was thirteen, and I was crying on the lounge room couch and she was ironing and pretending not to notice. She suddenly slammed down the iron and said, 'Look, you're not the only one who's miserable, you know. Sometimes you just have to put up with the bad things in life.' This was quite a breakthrough for my mother, because she never usually acknowledged the bad things at all. I said to her: 'Why does Dad always have to spoil things? I hate him.' She gave me this funny look over the ironing table. Then she told me, in this very calm, matter-of-fact voice, that our father was rotten to the core and had cheated on her all their married life. This was a real shock to me. It might sound really dumb, but I hadn't thought about him in that way before. I didn't really want to know that, you know? I was only a kid.

But normally, our mother hated anyone to make a fuss. You just got on with life. There was nothing that couldn't be fixed with a disprin and an early night and eventually the problem, whatever it was, would become one of our funny little stories. Something to laugh about at Christmas with our uncle and auntie.

The good thing about Melbourne was that our father had a job where he travelled a lot and he was away for most of every week, which meant the fighting and the rows died down. Or maybe they just got tired, I don't know. I started high school, it was a huge school, my first day was hideous. There were over 300 kids in my year and I didn't know a soul. I was the only one there with both parents with me. That was part of the image, always. She always got Dad to the school stuff. I don't know how she did it, but there he would be, in his colour-coordinated shirts and ties and his brand-name sunnies and his moussed hair. And there she would be at his side, smiling, smart suit, stiletto heels, incredibly out of date but *nice* – so that all the teachers thought what a lovely couple they were and what nice parents I had.

Edward was no help. He was a new boy too, and a nerd as well, but I never saw him. He never had many friends, anyway. He was never popular, like me.

I could never be like Edward. I have to have lots of people around me, you know? I like company. I get very bored on my own. Dad always said that's when I always got into the most trouble. He was wrong. Once I started high school, my friends and I got into heaps of really serious trouble when we were all together. We were BAD!'

'WHAT SORT OF KID WOULD ... ?'

Every sort of kid.

Young people who have been neglected by their families, tossed aside by society and preyed upon by those they trusted commit or attempt suicide; boy and girls from devoted, loving homes do it too.

So do the young men and women who find themselves in categories somewhere in between. More than ten percent of young people in Australia attempt suicide at least once during their youth.

Youth suicide can occur in the best and worst of families. In the end it depends on each individual young person and how effectively they have been immunised by their parents, their relatives, their peers, their teachers, and their friends against this modern day epidemic of self-destruction. It depends on their ability to cope with the realities of life – the degree of hopelessness and helplessness they feel when things are going wrong. It depends on the amount of alcohol they drink and how much marijuana they are smoking. Perhaps it even depends on that old cliche – their fighting spirit.

WHO IS AT RISK?

The resilience of young people to the crises and stresses of their lives varies enormously. As neglected as they appear to be, broken kids are sometimes more resilient than their lovingly protected peers. On the other hand, when children have been robbed of their self-esteem through poverty, abuse and cruelty, some of them see no real reason to hang around in a world which promises more of the same.

When it comes to anxiety young people are no different to everyone else. They have a lot to worry about – for a whole range of reasons. There are examinations to pass, there is the problem of finding a job in an economic climate where full-time workers are putting in longer and longer hours to keep ahead of the competition, and even fifty-year-old fathers are not sure how soon they may be thrown on the scrap heap. There can be changes within the family (remarriage, new children, older siblings leaving home, illness), and other changes like long-term unemployment and poverty, created by the outside world but having their biggest effect behind closed doors. They may experience loss (family breakdown after divorce, death, illness, moving away) or the stress of maintaining relationships with family and friends. Add the future of the world and the monolithic struggle to save the environment from destruction and it makes quite an impressive list of things to worry about, especially when whether they are meek or not, they are part of the generation that will soon inherit the earth.

Inevitably, teenagers and young men and women in their early twenties, all of them on the threshold of adult life, cope with stress, change and responsibility in many different ways. What will be devastating for one will be no big deal for another.

But there are some crucial differences between all young people and adult men and women.

Adolescents judge themselves very harshly and constantly compare themselves with their peers. They usually recognise only black-and-white choices and although time is on their side, they are impatient for solutions. They are intensely sensitive to rejection and failure. Rarely do they have the experience and maturity to see their troubles in perspective. That's what makes them rather difficult to live with, even if they are happy, healthy and, from an adult's perspective, relatively free of care.

Adolescents take risks. How dangerous these risks become depend on whether they are trying prove their growing independence or whether their circumstances mean a state of drugged oblivion is preferable to waking up each morning and facing the future.

Excessive drinking and drug taking (particularly marijuana smoking) leads to mental illness. Alcohol and marijuana work on the brain in different ways but they are both powerful players in the tragedy of youth suicide.

Unfortunately, adolescents are not usually inclined to discuss problems with their parents. They yearn for independence but how can they be independent if they run to their mum with every little worry in their life, if their dad takes over each time they hit a hump? Their friends become very important to them, although some of the issues which are troubling them are not the sort of thing they want to admit to their peers.

Even when they do approach their parents, the generation which grew up in the post-war years may be unable to provide any answers. Their own jobs may be in jeopardy. They, too, drink to ease the pain, even if they have learned the wisdom of moderation. They may have smoked dope in the sixties and seventies – it was five to fifty percent less potent than the stuff kids are smoking now, but maybe it's hypocritical to recommend abstinence to their children ... *(Really? Then why does everyone agree that lives have been saved by the introduction of drink-driving laws and seat belts; why isn't anyone suggesting that it's hypocritical to make sure our kids don't take the same risks we did on the roads?)*

From the age of about fifteen, life gets as complicated as a quilt in which half the squares in the once precise patchwork have come unstitched. There's so much you want to do and adults are hitting you with a multitude of new expectations but at the same time as they demand that you prove yourself responsible they put up barriers to keep you out of their world. You can't do this, you can't have that, surely you are not going out in public looking like *that*, you can't be the person you really are – but who *is* the person you really are? Sometimes it's just all too much.

PARTICULARLY IF . . .

. . . Particularly if you're terrified that your mum and dad are going to break up. All those rows and those long cold silences when you come in – do they think you're deaf and dumb or just stupid? Who would you live with if they split? What if they made you choose? You love them both, boring and batty as they are. What if the one you went with moved away and you had to leave all your friends? What if they married somebody else, somebody you hate, like that slime ball Mum sometimes brings home from work who looks at you as if you were a soft centre chocolate and he was peeling off the wrapping? What if neither of them wanted you, if they both wanted to make a fresh start? Where would you go? What would you do?

. . . Particularly if you've always been a bad kid, right from when you bit the other boys at playgroup, and all through primary school, when you spent most of your time outside the principal's office and definitely in high school where you hold the record for suspensions. School work is too hard and you'd rather be a clown in class than make a fool of yourself by taking education seriously. Trouble is your middle name, nothing ever works out right for you, even when you try. There's a whole profession of counsellors out there who have been trained to help kids like you but none of them have ever come up with anything except the fact that you have a 'conduct disorder' – which is pretty fucking obvious and which you don't need a university degree to work out.

...Particularly if you are a boy who is attracted to boys. It's all supposed to be okay these days and they even have the Mardi Gras on the TV ... you've made some interesting friends on the Internet who say it's fine, it's the way you're born, it's normal ... but if Mum or Dad knew they'd die. Anyway, perhaps you're not. Maybe Mum was right the other day when she said it was people who should know better leading unhappy kids astray. It's just that the way you felt when you were with Simon was so different ... and let's face it, kissing Linda was an endurance test ... like rubbing your lips through slush ... whereas with Simon ... but what sort of life would you have ... with AIDS and everything ... nothing but fear and revolting stuff in men's toilets ... and the old man would probably kill you ... anyway, it's hardly the sort of thing you're going to tell anyone around here.

...Particularly if you don't much like yourself. Your body is all wrong, too thin or too fat, too big or too small, your skin is like pizza or else it's the colour of spaghetti which is supposed to be a good thing, only tell that to the gorgeous guys with tans; your hair won't grow the way everyone else's does, the clothes that look so cool in the shops and on your friends make you look like a garbage bag. Not that you can afford any of the best brands anyway. Or maybe it's not so much your physical appearance that makes you ashamed as your bumbling brain, your inability to understand what they're getting at in English or Maths, when so many other kids seem to take being smart for granted. The teachers treat you like a moron so you behave like one; shit, they're probably right. Why did you end up with mush for brains when other kids were given the real thing?

...Particularly when you're drinking heavily or regularly smoking marijuana and your peers are all doing it too because it's cool. The bliss that pot provides feels good at the time and numbs the pain you've been feeling but you're never happy without it and maybe that's not such a good thing. Someone told you that grog and pot are guaranteed to trash your system and very likely to stuff up your energy, your ideas, your appearance and your ambition. (*What* ambition?) It now turns out that the effects of dope on your brain can be really bloody dangerous. But even if you believe all this, how likely are your mates to listen to shit like that?

...Particularly if your mum (or dad, or sister or brother or beloved gran) has died and everyone has stopped feeling sorry for you and they seem to expect you to be getting on with things without realising that you still miss her so much that even the faint, sweet smell that still lingers in the bedroom cupboard brings stinging tears to your eyes and makes your throat ache. What's the point in doing all the study and 'making something of yourself' when she won't be around to see it happen; why decorate for Christmas when there's so much sadness in the world; why watch television comedies when nobody smiles at home any more; why not be with her? She's left you alone – if you were with her you wouldn't be so alone.

That's hardly the sort of stuff you could say to a friend. On the other hand, you can't say it to Dad or the rest of the family either, because they're still hurting too. Or so they say.

...Particularly if someone you all know, a good friend, perhaps even a member of your own or a close friend's family, has committed suicide, and you're wondering why and where they are now and whether it's a solution for you. And you're scared, terrified in fact, that it might be, and you don't want it to be, and you wish desperately there was someone you could tell. But who?

...Particularly if your mates are too far away, gone to the towns looking for work and you are stuck in this rural backwater where the only entertainment is watching the dogs mate. The farm's going broke and there's no future in farming, no hope at all, you can see it in your father's blank stare when he comes home Fridays from the job he found at the factory 300 kilometres away and you can see it in the slope of your mother's shoulders as she sits on the tractor and you keep thinking about the guns under the stairs and maybe going roo shooting and maybe just finishing it all, except that Mum can barely cope now and without you she'd be history.

...Particularly if you are a dark-skinned indigenous Australian living in your own country among people whose history and culture has swamped your own; who have caught you, confused you, castigated and abused you and finally, not knowing what to do with you, have demanded that you show some independence of spirit and cast you adrift in the changing tides of a society which after only 200 years seems to have lost direction.

...Particularly if your parents have come to Australia from another country and the differences in the way they want you to live and the way you and your peers expect you to spend your time are wider than the ocean they crossed to get here. If your mates knew how different it was at your place, they'd crack up – *how* embarrassing. How do you keep your home life secret? Lisa called it 'Home and Away' – like living in two worlds. Lisa was the only one you could talk to about it; she understood. Or so you thought. And now she's dropped you. She's just like the others, laughing at you behind your back, whispering secrets around their hands. You told her you loved her and now she's probably telling them everything and you have no one to talk to, nobody who understands, nobody to trust.

...Particularly if you are a child who lives, more often than not, on the streets of a city that neither cares nor cries for you. There's no point in talking about it; your mates are in the same situation as you – maybe worse. They are the runaways who have rejected or been rejected by those to whom they once belonged; broken adolescents from broken homes, unloved, unwanted, neglected, ignorant of their worth.

...Particularly if you have been physically hurt, sexually abused or emotionally damaged by those who were meant to protect you. If even your dad doesn't love you, what is your life worth? It must be your fault – otherwise why doesn't Mum make him stop? The suffering you are now doing is the punishment for your crime. What crime? Just being here you suppose. But there's something you can do about that. Unless somebody cares enough to stop you.

Somebody like who?

DROPPING THEIR BUNDLE

Many young people take a gamble and talk to their friends about their unhappiness. When the situation is serious, few kids know how to help. Frequently they are sworn to secrecy. It's a pact that's often fatal. When it comes to suicide, the reward for loyalty is the loss of a friend.

None of this means that all young people who are anxious about their relationships within their families, their friends, their physical appearance, their academic ability, their job prospects, their sexuality, their sex life (or lack of it) or any of the other multitude of subjects which can preoccupy the adolescent mind, are likely to try to die.

Rarely does a single issue or problem cause a young person to take their life. It's common but very misleading to assume that a boy committed suicide because he mucked up his exams, or because he didn't get into medicine at university, or because he lost his job; or that a girl attempted to kill herself because her boyfriend broke off their relationship or because her father and mother decided to get a divorce.

It's never that easy. Almost always, a suicidal state of mind is the result of an accumulation of troubles and attitudes which probably began in childhood. There may be a catalyst, the proverbial straw that sends the camel crashing to the ground under his agonising burden, but the real problem is the burden itself, a whole load of problems and distress which finally becomes too heavy because the young person has never found a way to off-load or cope with any of them.

When a young man shoots himself, said one researcher, the gun has probably been cocked since the boy was three years old.

Thousands of teenagers are prone to depression. Too much depression, left too long untreated, can result in the anger, lethargy, sadness and unbearable hopelessness which may convince young people that life is not worth hanging around for – that leaving early is a solution to their pain.

'DEPRESSION? WHAT HAVE THEY GOT TO BE MISERABLE ABOUT?'

It was Carol, a woman with tired eyes and a blue dress, who stood up at the Class of '65 Reunion Party and said: 'My greatest achievement is that I live in the same house as my five teenage children'.

She was given a standing ovation.

Firmly entrenched in the minds of parents who were adolescents in the sixties is the conception that having teenage children is an endurance test of massive proportions. During the past thirty years we have all become convinced that pimples, periods and parties, booze, dreadful clothes, alarming hair, body piercing, drugs, sex and the constant battle for independence is as unpleasantly inevitable as supermarket queues, traffic congestion and computerised banking.

With powerful media and marketing forces baying at their hugely upholstered heels, today's teenagers are pilloried, categorised and catastrophised within an inch of their lives.

No wonder they are depressed.

Young people are everywhere. They are on the streets, in the shops, on trains and buses and beaches, pouring out of schools and ambling around universities. They laugh, they talk, they call out loudly and tease their friends. They giggle, they sulk a little, they smile. They stick together.

Where do all these kids turn into the monstrous problem children we hear so much about? Is it in the hell holes which were once simple suburban bedrooms that this transition takes place? Do their personalities undergo some sort of cerebral revolution as they lie prone in front of the television with their feet on the coffee table for which you sold your youngest child's soul? Are all of them really so awful?

Behind closed doors, on the other side of the treated pine fences, the majority of young people live with their families. And believe it or not, most of them, most of the time, rub along quite well with the people who love them. Which begs the question: is their transition into maturity as melodramatic and maddening as the popular image of the teenager suggests?

Adolescence is a time of change, of trying new experiences, of developing independence. Since the beginning of time, young people in their teens have gradually broken free from the protection of their families and tested their own survival skills.

Throughout the centuries, children have looked forward to that time. So have their proud parents. At Jewish Bar Mitzvahs, at Aboriginal initiation ceremonies, at the grand debutante balls which some Australian communities continue to enjoy, the transition from childhood to adult life has always been regarded as an occasion for celebration. The difference today is that instead of welcoming adolescence, or attaching special significance to traditional customs and rituals, the vast majority of parents simply dread their children's teenage years.

Adults who expect drama and trouble tend to get it. The kids know what is expected of them. They see it on the screen, they read about it every day in newspapers and magazines. They hear themselves discussed in disagreeable detail. They are going through a tumultuous time; they are expected to be thoughtless, rude, aggressive, selfish, untidy, easily upset, frequently depressed and alienated from the rest of society. So a lot of them are – particularly if nobody at home wants to talk to them about their feelings or listen to what they have to say.

The other big difference today is that the new ultra-sensitive, caring, quality-time-worshipping parents no longer put a stop to unacceptably bad or selfish behaviour. Convinced that it is inevitable, they put up with it in the name of tolerance whereas the truth is that they almost always have too many other things to do – and anything is better than wrangling with an adolescent.

Especially one who is taller than they are.

Many mums and dads allow themselves to believe that the troubles of adolescence will gradually pass. They submit to the rubbery image of Everyone Else's Parents and standards which were never theirs. Frazzled, frustrated and frantically busy, many parents make up for the lack of time they spend with their teenagers by providing them with material possessions and driving them to casual jobs where they can earn the cash they need to make them happy. Meanwhile they are depriving their young people of the most valuable gifts of all – the discipline that shows how much they care and the time that every adolescent needs.

An insidious danger is emerging from the popular conception of normal adolescence as a period of trauma and trouble. The danger is that genuine depression in young people is going unnoticed until it is too late.

TRULY MADLY DEEPLY SAD

It is possible to feel sad without being ill with depression. On the other hand, it is impossible to be depressed without feeling sad.

Depression is linked to a majority of youth suicides. It is even more closely linked to suicide attempts – for every death there are many more young people who try to kill themselves. But how do you tell if a young person is seriously depressed? What is the difference between mental illness, depression and simple sadness?

Symptoms of depression in young people may include recurring sadness or volatile moods, feelings of helplessness and hopelessness, irritability, withdrawal, persistent boredom, low energy, poor concentration, changes in eating or sleep patterns, deteriorating school performance, increased risk taking and frequent complaints of physical illness. This may sound like a description of any average adolescent on a bad day, but when any of these symptoms are persistent or prolonged, it is dangerous to assume that it's all just part of growing up.

One big difference between adult and adolescent depression is that many young people appear to be angry rather than down or sad. Perhaps friends who know them really well recognise that they are unhappy, but what most people see is a young person who pushes people away, who plays up, behaves badly and takes dangerous risks. Not unnaturally, the first instinct of most adults is to leave them alone.

Those seriously at risk of damaging themselves as a result of depression include young people who have already attempted suicide, who are suffering from psychiatric disorders, who abuse alcohol and drugs, who are grieving and who may be experiencing serious family problems.

Adolescents tend to be impulsive. One minute they're fed up to here and the next minute they're taking action to finish their life. Sometimes there's such a short period of time between a crisis and the act. If depression recurs frequently and is not noticed, discussed or treated, it can be very serious. The high rate of suicide among young people is frightening proof that depression can kill.

Some figures indicate that as many as ninety percent of young people who suicide have some history of mental health problems. In most cases, this means they were suffering from depression.

The scariest question of all is: what was wrong with the remaining ten percent?

SICK IN THE HEAD?

Perhaps the two most terrifying illnesses that cast a shadow over modern society are mental illness and cancer. Cancer threatens our lives; many people still regard it as a death sentence. Mental illness threatens our sanity; millions of people believe anyone who is 'sick in the head' is crazy rather than ill.

There are many different forms and degrees of mental illness, just as there are many different forms and degrees of cancer. Like cancer, some forms of mental illness, if caught early, can be totally cured. Like cancer, mental illness may recur, only to be beaten back again. Like cancer, mental illness neglected and left to grow out of control may result in death.

There's a stigma attached to mental illness that goes way back to the dark ages when madness was linked with the devil, when craziness was connected with evil. In our enlightened age we have dispensed with the devil in almost all his forms, yet we are still frightened and ashamed of mental illness, particularly if it affects a member of our family.

On the other hand, while depression is the most common form of mental illness, few people believe it's an illness at all. It's more likely to be regarded as a weakness, a failure of the person concerned to come to terms with the reality of life.

Medical research is now attempting to turn this attitude around. The health profession has recognised that depression can be an enormous handicap. The World Health

Organization is currently investigating the number of years lost through disabilities resulting from illness. As a disabling illness, depression is at the top of the table and is predicted to become much worse.

Depression is a condition which sets in when people are young and, while they may not be dying of it in droves, it has a huge impact on their employment and economic prospects, on their social life, their relationships, their quality of life.

HOW DO THEY GET IT?

Dr George Patton is an Associate Professor in Adolescent Psychiatry with the Department of Paediatrics and Psychiatry at the University of Melbourne, who has been conducting research into depression in young people for several years. According to Dr Patton, it was believed for a long time that mental disorders of any kind did not occur in children or adolescents until they reached their twenties. Not until the early 1900s was it established that certain mental disorders, including some forms of melancholia or depression, could begin before the age of twenty.

The two best-known, severely disabling forms of mental illness are schizophrenia and manic depression. These are called *bipolar* conditions. Symptoms can show up even before the age of ten and certainly in adolescence.

Depression, which is a *unipolar* condition, is recognised less easily, especially in teenagers.

The current popular assumptions about teenage turmoil were developed early this century, when some psychiatrists argued that adolescence was an evolutionary process during which human beings moved from a very fundamental type of thinking to a more sophisticated cognitive development. 'This process was associated with significant emotional upheaval,' said Dr Patton. 'Young people were expected to experience emotional turmoil as a normal part of growing into maturity – if not, they would end up repressed.

'Nobody believed that depression in adolescence would have an impact on adult lives; it was just part of working through the problems of youth.'

As appealing as these notions were, and despite the huge numbers of people who still believe all young people get 'puberty blues' which will fade in the normal course of time, the theory doesn't stand up.

'First,' said Dr Patton, 'it does not appear that all adolescents go through a period of significant emotional turmoil. Sure, there are probably more changes at this time of life than at any other. However, if you look at the extent to which a large proportion of adolescents experience alienation, distress and emotional upheaval, you can see that only about twenty percent are affected. It's not universal in any way.

'It now seems there is a lot more continuity between adult and adolescent problems than was previously thought. It really looks as if we have to treat chronic adolescent depression much more seriously.'

WHAT'S ACTUALLY WRONG WITH THEM?

If you are a businessman with corporate pressures pinning you to your desk, deadlines to meet and a family to keep; if you are the mother of young children who seem to tie you interminably to the washing machine and the microwave; if your elderly parents are desperately in need of you but so is everyone else; if your husband is out of work and there are birthdays coming and no money for petrol let alone presents … it's impossible to understand how or why a young person on the threshold of life could be seriously depressed.

According to the National Health and Medical Research Council's (NHMRC) *Depression in young people: clinical practice guidelines*, (1997), there are three types of depression from which adolescents and young people are likely to suffer.

The first is 'depressed mood', in which those affected feel unhappy for an unspecified period of time. Up to two-fifths of young people in the community suffer from depressed mood in any six-month period.

The second is 'depressive syndrome', referring to a series of depressive and other emotional symptoms. Five percent of young people suffer from depressive syndrome.

The third is 'depressive disorders' or 'clinical depression' which refers to disturbances affecting emotional, behavioural and cognitive functioning. Clinical depression is usually diagnosed after psychiatric testing.

About a third of young people with a depressive disorder attempt suicide in the twenty years following this diagnosis and at least three percent commit suicide during this period.

RISK FACTORS

Some young people are more likely to get depressed than others. According to evidence presented to the NHMRC, the risk results from a combination of many symptoms, circumstances and situations.

Definite factors include:
- Anxiety, conduct disorder or substance abuse
- Being over fifteen
- Being female
- Having a depressed parent
- Having a previous history of depression

Probable factors include:
- Having a close biological relative with depression
- Exposure to stressful life events
- Being born late in the current century

Possible factors include:

- Poor self-esteem, negative thinking, dysfunctional attitudes
- Poor self-control or social competence
- Vulnerable personality, being neurotic
- Parents divorced, separated or in conflict
- Uncaring or over-controlling parental style during childhood
- Early childhood sexual and physical abuse
- Being of Aboriginal or Torres Strait Islander descent
- Residing in rural areas
- Learning difficulties
- Sleeping problems
- Being poor
- Poor peer relationships
- Decreasing school performance
- Having coexisting medical problems
- Being homeless or in custody
- Coming from a non-English speaking background
- Hormonal changes during puberty
- Parental death
- Attempting suicide

According to the NHMRC guidelines, the best deterrents to clinical depression in young people include good peer relationships in later adolescence, good relationships with parents and being employed.

Common sense tells us that young people who get on well with their friends and their parents are less likely to become deeply depressed. However, no matter how good the family relations are, there is strong evidence to suggest that if a parent or close relative suffers from chronic depression, or has a history of depressive illness, there is a risk of the son or daughter inheriting this condition.

Employment – or the lack of it – is a particularly serious problem for young men. Training for employment and holding down a job is a terrifically important factor in providing them with self-respect.

Now that there are so few jobs for the boys the worry is that that they are unmotivated, they have nowhere in life to go, they cannot plan ahead. Where do they get the status of being the provider, of achieving something for themselves, of being independent?

The risk of girls becoming depressed becomes higher following puberty. Dr Patton said this may be related to biological changes associated with the onset of periods, or psychological changes associated with new sexual and social roles.

STARTING YOUNG

Depression is a mystifying illness because what some people will see as massive barriers which set them back and cause debilitating depression, others will regard as hurdles which can be vaulted and left behind.

Dr Patton's work with adolescents indicates that depression does not develop overnight. Almost universally, young people who become depressed have been showing signs of mild depression from an early age – they may have been unhappy or anxious children, easily tired and prone to irritability; for months or even years they may have been having trouble with sleep and concentration, losing their confidence, feeling low about themselves.

'These kids have not been ill but something has not been quite right,' said Dr Patton. 'Most of them do not go on to become clinically depressed, but a sufficient number of them do to indicate that help is needed.'

Dr Patton estimated that in a majority of cases, early intervention could have prevented minor depressive symptoms from developing into worsening depressive disorders.

This doesn't mean seeing a psychiatrist – probably not even a doctor. It could be an understanding parent, a sympathetic school teacher, a counsellor, or a friend who talks the young person into a more positive frame of mind. 'It may be that it will just pass but for that to happen the sadness that is affecting their lives must be taken seriously from the beginning,' said Dr Patton.

IS THERE SOMETHING THEY CAN TAKE FOR IT?

If young people are going to drop out of school, fail their exams, lose their friends or do themselves some harm through binge drinking – then it's time to take action. When the symptoms of depression are continual and show no sign of diminishing, or when a young person is significantly handicapped by their depression in their day-to-day life, clinical treatment is required.

This can be in the form of medication or psychological counselling or a combination of both. It's essential that families, doctors and health workers – and if possible, the young person's close friends as well – work together to defeat the demons of depression.

Professional counsellors tend to look at the young person's situation – their school, home and social life. When treating depression, their aim is to build up the person's positive regard for themselves. Talking about their problems is useful but young people should also be persuaded to do things which give them a sense of achievement.

There is a lot of resistance to prescribing antidepressant medication for young people and no evidence that medication makes a long-term difference.

'Treating them psychologically is preferable,' said Dr Patton, 'because there is a prospect of lasting change. While medication will work while they are taking it, unless there is a corresponding change in their social life or in a psychological context, it's unlikely that medication is going to be effective in the long term.'

Antidepressant medication influences the way messages are carried in the brain – it reverses disturbances in the neurotransmitters – or 'nerve pathways' – which affect people's thoughts and to some extent, their behaviour.

Specific studies have not been done on adolescents taking antidepressants and to what extent this affects them over the long term. The traditional antidepressants are called tricyclics and are suitable, said Dr Patton, for people with a melancholic disposition but no desire to do themselves harm. A new group of antidepressants is now the preferred option for doctors treating adolescents with depression. These are called serotonin selective reuptake inhibitors (SSRI's); as the name suggests they have an effect on the chemical serotonin, which is found in the brain. Common trade names for these antidepressants include Prozac, Erocap, Lovan, Zactin, Aropax and Luvox.

The advantage of these is that they are less dangerous if taken in excessive amounts. 'However,' said Dr Patton, 'young people can't stay on them forever. They are useful in getting people through a critical situation, in getting them functioning again. Ideally we should then look at the other circumstances of their lives so that they do not need to rely on the medication in the future.'

The third and least attractive option for treating depression in young people is hospitalisation. Because of the dearth of suitable facilities, this is only likely to be recommended if the young person is under serious threat of death from suicide, self-injury or reduced eating and drinking. It may be suggested in cases where the young person requires basic care and support that is unavailable at home or where the depression is severe and unresponsive to treatment.

IS SEROTONIN TO BLAME?

Medical science has recently revealed that a catalyst which causes a depressed person to take their life may be a physical rather than a mental or emotional one. Autopsy studies have revealed that many people who have committed suicide have very low levels of serotonin in their brain.

New research suggests that low levels of this chemical may be the reason why some young people decide to die while others struggle on.

Dr Sheila Clark, a South Australian general practitioner and author of *After Suicide: Help for the Bereaved* who has been working in the area of support for those bereaved by suicide for the past ten years, explained that the brain is made of many nerve cells.

'Thought processes are created by micro-electrical impulses passing along a series of these nerve cells,' said Dr Clark. 'Between each of these cells is a gap. When the impulse reaches the end of a nerve cell, this cell then sends out a little jet of serotonin to stimulate an impulse in the next cell, and so on.

'According to the autopsy studies, low serotonin levels have been found following suicide in people who suffered depression, schizophrenia and even after impulsive or apparently "spontaneous" suicides.'

Researchers have also identified the fact that the centre of the brain where serotonin levels were registering as low is adjacent to that area of the brain which regulates inhibitive behaviour. This could mean that a person in despair is more likely to take that last fatal step if their brain's 'stop and think' button is not getting the stimulation it needs to function correctly.

'With diabetes, the body does not produce adequate amounts of insulin so it can't manipulate its sugar levels,' said Dr Clark. 'In this case the brain does not produce adequate serotonin, so it has difficulty controlling thoughts. Because it is a physical condition over which nobody has any control, the knowledge that the person they have lost was suffering from low serotonin levels can be immeasurably helpful to bereaved families. It provides a no-fault, no stigma explanation for why the person took their own life.'

Medical science now needs to find out more about the control of serotonin and effective ways of raising its levels. One theory is that severe stress decreases serotonin. It is also possible that genetics might play a part in the fact that some people are more susceptible to low levels of serotonin than others.

So what is 'normal'?

The majority of young people who are suffering from depression receive no treatment for their problem.

Most young men suffering from depression don't even talk about it. By the time they reach adolescence they have been well schooled in the Australian way of masculinity – keeping their troubles and anxieties deep within themselves while presenting an image of tough courage to their friends and families. Psychotherapist Steve Biddulph claims in his book *Manhood* that boys and young men are destined for a lifetime of unhappiness unless society allows them to escape from the loneliness, compulsive competition and emotional timidity which is caging them into a false and unnatural role.

Adults tend to ignore their children's depression, or perhaps they don't notice it at all. This is mainly due to the misconception that depression, like acne, is normal in adolescence. It can also be attributed to the enormous range of symptoms of depression and young people's ability and desire to mask their true feelings.

There is a drastic lack of appropriate facilities for assessing and treating young people, inadequate continuity of care and the problem of kids with attitude – they don't want, seek or know about getting help for the way they feel.

They know they're normal. They've seen 'The Simpsons'.

'I think there's a lot of scope for doing things a lot better,' said Dr Patton. 'We don't know yet if early intervention works with adolescent depression. The development of accessible effective psychiatric services for adolescents is only just beginning.'

Young people tend to get lost in the health system; neither small and vulnerable nor independent and fully grown, they fall into a valley somewhere between the already rocky range of adults' and children's services. Only very recently has the need for specialist youth services been acknowledged.

What have they got to be miserable about?
Heaps.

SOFT POISON

There's nothing like a big long drag on a marijuana bong to convince you that life is not as bad as it was half an hour ago.

And there's nothing like a big fat bag of marijuana in your brain to convince you that the only way you can not worry and be happy is to keep on smoking dope until your mind gets used to the idea that this is the way it's always going to be.

Which is why most of the kids who kill themselves have been regularly smoking what is so insidiously sold to a still-trusting public as 'the soft drug'.

Of twenty young people whose families were interviewed in depth for this book, nineteen had been smoking marijuana prior to their death. Many had been regularly drinking alcohol as well. Of the hundreds of others who make up the sad statistics, many had used marijuana at some stage of their short lives.

They had all believed the hype and so had many of their parents – that pot is nowhere near as harmful as cigarettes and probably less dangerous than grog.

Like many of Australia's middle-aged and misled millions ('I used it so why shouldn't my kid?') and their glazed and damaged children, they were misinformed.

HARD FACTS ABOUT THE SOFT DRUG

John Anderson is a psychophysiologist. He examines human behaviour by studying the way the brain reacts to how human beings behave. His research for the past few years has centred on the effects of drugs on brain function.

John Anderson admits that he, too, used marijuana in his youth, but unlike many others, he doesn't want the kids using it. He has learned things about dope smoking that the people who want to legalise marijuana are taking great pains to ignore.

'Marijuana is the most frightening of all the drugs I have studied,' he said. 'The potential harm it can do in the long term is far more dangerous than heroin, ecstasy or any of the other illicit substances.

'Because it is fat soluble, marijuana stays in the system for at least a month; it clogs the fat glands of the brain for months if not years. Other drugs, and alcohol in particular, are quickly excreted. Alcohol is fully water soluble, although it is much more potent than pot at the time of ingestion.

'Initially, marijuana increases the flow of blood to the brain, creating the anticipated "high". Blood flow is important because it carries oxygen to the brain and oxygen is what our brains need to function efficiently.

'Within about half an hour, the blood flow rapidly decreases by about twenty percent below normal levels. The smoker feels rotten again – so he or she has another joint. Up goes the blood flow, down it comes again, and so it goes on.

'In the end they become constantly depressed unless they are stoned. That doesn't seem to work as well for them any more so they may decide to try something stronger. They get hold of some speed, or some other amphetamine or hallucinogen, which is probably mixed with rubbish which does them even more harm – let's face it, the people who are selling these substances are not interested in quality control.'

Regular use of marijuana can decrease blood flow by up to twenty percent. According to John Anderson, even a four percent decrease in the flow of blood to the brain is a significant problem. People who are permanently incapacitated with that dreaded affliction of old age, Alzheimers disease, often have as little as four percent decrease in blood flow in specific regions of the brain.

'The main problem with marijuana,' he said, 'is that it decreases blood flow throughout the whole brain. All the parts of the brain are affected, which is why people's moods swing, their memories give out and even their music sounds different to them.'

Most people already know that when people with schizophrenia or Attention Deficit Disorder (ADD) use marijuana, it makes their condition much worse. Unfortunately, they often do use it, because they want a temporary reprieve from their feelings of depression and other disabling symptoms. People with these conditions make up sixteen percent of our total youth population.

When marijuana is used by people who do *not* have schizophrenia or ADD – that is, young men and women who do not have a mental or neurological disorder – the 'soft' drug creates a level of brain dysfunction that is the same as if they had been born with schizophrenia or ADD. 'In fact, people with schizophrenia and ADD usually have an eight to twelve percent decrease in blood flow, while people who smoke dope regularly for a month have a fifteen to twenty percent decrease in blood flow to the brain,' said John Anderson.

The result is that they become lethargic, less articulate (having a problem finding words to finish their sentences) and paranoid (they frequently get obsessed about getting caught); most seriously, they are predisposed to long term chronic depression which can make them very angry, both with themselves and with the world.

'Another thing that marijuana does is to confuse the information that is getting to the brain,' said John Anderson.

'Marijuana affects the signals the brain receives, so it's much harder to work things out. People with ADD get their brain signals too fast. People with schizophrenia get their signals too slowly. Because marijuana initially speeds up the signals, then as blood flow reduces, slows the signals down, it has a particularly dangerous effect on people already suffering from schizophrenia – their psychosis often leads them to suicide. In otherwise well people, it distorts perception and interferes with the electrical activity and neurotransmitters of the brain, creating an artificial form of schizophrenia.'

One in ten people who have a drug-induced psychosis commits suicide.

The effects of marijuana on normal people are short term, said John Anderson. Depending on the frequency and amount of marijuana they have been using, it takes from six to ninety days for the system to rid itself of the effects of the drug. Continued usage, however, eventually results in the brain remaining damaged.

Not all youth suicides occur after long-term depression. Sometimes suicide will result from reduced impulse control. 'People who are stoned are more likely than others to act on impulse,' said John Anderson, 'because their brains have been getting confused signals.'

The effect of alcohol on the brain is a totally different process but makes marijuana-induced depression worse. Alcohol and marijuana are both major contributors to youth suicide. The tragedy is that a lot of kids are using both, some are supplementing these with other drugs as well. All those young brains out there don't know what is going on.

Ignorance is bad enough; politics are worse. If the pro-legalisation lobby succeeds in decriminalising marijuana use, it's inevitable that the incidence of drug-induced depression will become widespread in this country.

'The situation will be the same as it is now with cigarettes,' said John Anderson. 'People will die from the diseases these drugs cause but the government will make billions of dollars out of it.'

The vast majority of young people are not aware that one way or another, their favourite drugs may be softly poisoning them to death.

COUNTRY KIDS: WHO CARES?

It's quiet out in the paddocks. You don't have to talk much. There's just the grass, seas of it, yellowing under the parching sun and crackling under your boots. There are the animals. You can talk to the animals, but they won't listen.

It's quiet out in the paddocks. You don't have to talk at all. You don't have to think either, if you don't want to. Anyway, what is there to think about? Dad? Always angry, all tied up inside like a coil of rusty wire, useless, knotted, no work, no money to feed the family. Mum? Tight lipped, never smiling no more, doing blokes work half the time while the old man sits with a bottle in his hand, waiting for a job to jump up and bite him on the boot. Kath? Sulking and whining for new clothes when she knows there's no cash. Clinging to that young kid she says is her boyfriend, winding herself all over him even though he calls her a slut to her face. Smoking dope till she's silly as a headless chook. Next thing she'll have something in the oven – and it won't be chicken, that's for sure.

Where's it all going to end? The farm's going to go. The family's going to go. Shit, everything's going.

It's quiet out in the paddocks. You don't have to talk. You don't have to think, not ever again, if you don't want to. The gun's in the ute, behind the seat. You might shoot a wild pig. Anyhow, who cares?

There is one group of young men who get no help when they need it, who probably don't even know they need help and who never draw attention to themselves. They are the country kids, the boys from the bush, about whom we hear nothing until they are dead. When you analyse their lives, this should come as no surprise.

The rate of suicide among young men in country areas has increased more than fifty percent since 1986. According to the Australian Bureau of Statistics in 1992, among rural males aged fifteen to twenty-four, there were 37.7 suicide deaths for every 100,000 people, compared with 24.7 per 100,000 in urban areas. In contrast, official statistics show a very slightly lower rate of suicide deaths among young females in rural areas – 5.4 compared with 5.7 in urban districts. (*Youth Suicide in Australia*, 1995).

Dr Michael Dudley, a child and adolescent psychiatrist at the Prince of Wales Hospital, Sydney, has been conducting research into youth suicide generally and into rural youth suicide in particular.

Studies by Dr Dudley and his colleagues found that from 1964 to 1993 the suicide rate for young people doubled in metropolitan areas and trebled in towns with populations over 4,000. In towns with less than 4,000 people, the youth suicide rate increased by ten times.

In both the city and the country, young men are killing themselves in far greater numbers than young women. 'The rate at which young men are suiciding in cities has gone up by two-and-a-half times but in remote and rural areas the rate has increased about twelve times in young males aged fifteen to twenty-four,' said Dr Dudley.

'Female rates have remained fairly static, except in small rural areas where they are six times greater than ten years ago.'

In country areas throughout Australia, generations of families are being forced off the land because of falling incomes and economic failure; men, women and children are losing a lifestyle they had expected to go on into future generations.

Because of the economic slump in rural areas and the resulting unemployment situation, small towns are closing down; it seems as if everyone is going to the cities. The ratio of rural/urban suicides has remained the same for the last thirty years, but while country populations have dwindled, the numbers of deaths have not.

Rural areas are more traditional than cities and have had to absorb a greater rate of change than urban areas in recent times. Far fewer students finish high school and go to university; families are being broken up by economic difficulties; many country communities are in trouble. For young people, the established order of life is being taken away.

Add to this a fragmented health service, the fear that everybody in town will find out if you seek medical or any other kind of help, a proximity to firearms, exposure to domestic violence, the influence of alcohol, and endless hours of thinking time – and the reasons why country kids are dying by their own hand become less hard to understand.

'To young rural men there are important issues at stake,' said Dr Dudley. 'Male identity is very important; they know that as men they are expected to be strong, resolute and unafraid. Country kids like to live up to the national stereotype – they still want to be Anzacs. There is this belief that men from the bush are the toughest; it's a myth we have always promoted. It makes for a complex story.'

For rural youth the same general factors which affect young people everywhere are compounded by these other local factors. Even if they realise they are suffering from depression, they are unlikely to recognise this as a form of mental illness; this sort of 'weakness' is seen as a moral failing. If they ring anyone for help they risk someone else listening in on the party line; they worry about everyone around knowing about their problems.

The few boys who have talked to teachers or school counsellors speak freely about knowing what to do with a gun; from childhood they have had contact with death. They shoot and skin animals. They're not frightened by blood. When they're ready, if they want to, they'll use the gun on themselves. Among young men in rural areas, gun deaths have increased sixfold over the past twenty-five years.

Not many of them are likely to thank God they are country boys. Feeling useless and hopeless, they are out of control of what is going on around them. They may play up at school – getting an education seems hardly worth it. To escape from their problems, many of them drink and smoke marijuana, unaware that this is likely to increase rather than decrease their growing depression.

Some of the men and women of country stock believe their kids just need a kick up the bum. Attention and care takes longer.

RURAL ACTION

As concern grows about the plight of young people in country areas, there has been an upsurge of interest in rural health and mental health in particular. A number of conferences have been organised by the Australian Rural Health Research Institute and the National Rural Health Alliance to find solutions to youth problems.

The Commonwealth Government is funding a major intervention project which is being trialed in five rural communities and a number of other programs have been scheduled to get under way during 1997.

At this point the main obstacle to the prevention of rural youth suicide is that not enough is known about the risks and causes which push young people out onto the barren plains of despair.

'We don't have enough evidence,' said Dr Dudley. 'Rural youth comprises about thirty percent of Australia's young population, but despite our findings and newly instituted programs, no published information exists which enables us to compare the mental health of rural and metropolitan youth.

'In the long term, with more proven research, we can beat at the doors of the bureaucrats and the policy makers and the funders and say: "This is what's happening and why. Now we can do something about it".'

In the short term, many rural communities are working out ways to respond to their own situations and circumstances. Dr Dudley said solutions tailored to specific local needs were more likely to be successful.

Effective solutions currently being tried in rural areas include:

- The green card – young people at risk are provided with a card on which there is a number they can ring if they need to talk to someone at any time.
- Support from nurses – staff in country hospitals are made aware that young people coming into the wards with drug or alcohol related problems, or even seemingly accidental injuries, may be at risk of suicide and are given appropriate guidance about how to deal with them.
- Continuity of care – the person who first speaks to a young person who has hurt himself or herself sees them again for follow-up treatment or counselling. (This can be done with trained volunteers.)
- Contracting – for some young men and women, knowing somebody cares enough to phone them is enough. Their counsellor makes a contract with them to call them every few hours if necessary, until the black mood has passed.
- Cognitive behavioural therapy – this is professional counselling dealing with self-esteem and stress;

unfortunately, counsellors in country areas are thin on the ground. Travel time and the expense of running cars to scattered settlements restricts the frequency of counselling sessions.

- Educating local doctors (when there *is* a local doctor) about the needs of young people in their area.
- Control of access to weapons – it has been proven that if firearms are locked up, the incidence of death decreases.

'When it comes to guns, availability is a crucial factor,' said Dr Dudley. 'People think that if you stop a kid once, they'll just go and do it some other way instead, but you have to remember that suicidal ideas are ambivalent and transient. Feelings can vary a great deal in a relatively short time. If the idea is blocked, it can be stopped.'

It's quiet out in the paddocks. Nobody there, nobody to talk to, nobody to listen. As usual. Nobody wants to know.
Anyhow, who cares?

'I THOUGHT THEY ONLY DID IT IF ...'

'How's the book going?' asked the lady at the stocking counter. 'What I heard is that the ones who do it are all schizo's.'

'The more they talk about it,' said the dinner guest loftily, 'the less they are likely to do it.'

'Some kids just want to die,' said the elderly gentleman. 'No balls. May as well let 'em. They're bound to do it anyway.'

'No,' said the writer, wanting to weep. 'None of that is true. It's not true at all.'

For hundreds of years, suicide has been surrounded by its own particular mythology, some of it merely inaccurate but much of it malignant in its potential to allow people to destroy themselves.

For centuries suicide was regarded by most churches as a sin. The bodies of those who took their own lives could not be buried on sacred ground. Their souls became the property of the devil who sentenced them to an eternity of burning in hell. Even in today's more tolerant religious communities, there are those who continue to believe that to take any life, even one's own, is to defy God's commandment.

In 1984 New South Wales became the last of the Australian states to repeal the law that made suicide an illegal act. Until then, survivors risked being charged with attempted murder – of themselves. It is still illegal to assist a person to complete a suicide, although even this situation has been confused by the debate about proposed changes to euthanasia laws.

(Euthanasia was legal for a short time, and in specific circumstances, in the Northern Territory in 1996–97.)

There are a number of myths about suicide which thousands of people believe. You hear them in the street, in the shops, in the corridors of offices – the mutterings and murmurings, the flotsam and jetsam of excuses and explanations which wash around those who are left behind.

DEADLY MYTHS

1. People who talk, write or think about suicide won't do it. They are just looking for attention.
   This is **wrong**.
   Suicide prevention educators believe that if this particular myth could be destroyed, the suicide rate in Australia would be halved. Research is showing that up to eighty percent of people contemplating suicide tell somebody. Some of the signs they give may be difficult to detect, but they will be there. You will remember them later. If help is not provided, if the cry is ignored, trivialised or not heard at all, the suicide may be carried out – if not now, then maybe next time.
   2. Talking openly about suicide may make a person do it.
   This is **wrong**.
   Too many people believe that mentioning the 'S' word will put the idea into the disturbed person's head or worse – it may push people over the edge.
   Happy people who may be experiencing an unhappy stage or situation do not contemplate suicide. Desperately depressed people have often already considered the option.
   When asking them if they are actually considering harming themselves you are likely to get one of three replies. The most terrifying reply is 'yes'. The other two are 'No, but I was' or 'Of course not'. Whatever the response may be, talking

sensitively to them about the way they feel is proof of how much you care. When people feel isolated, abandoned, rejected, hopeless and worthless, you can correct their belief that nobody cares about them by showing your concern.

3. Suicidal people are insane.

This is **wrong.**

The majority of young people who commit suicide are suffering from depression, but while depression is a form of mental illness, it is not madness.

(*See* Depression: what have they got to be miserable about? *on pages 60–74.*)

Sports champions have committed suicide this year – so have school captains, brilliant scholars, loud car buffs, sleek bike riders, party animals and drama queens. They are the young people who spark the common comment: 'But why? He/she had everything to live for'. Like their less distinguished peers, none of them were 'mad'; almost certainly most of them, for reasons of their own, were intensely sad. They all reached a point of despair which, at least on the day they died, took them beyond hope.

4. Suicidal people are determined to die; genuine attempts occur without any warning.

This is **wrong.**

Only a small proportion of suicidal people give no warning signs. The overwhelming majority don't want to die; they simply want to bring an end to their problems and the intense emotional pain they feel. They usually give clues to what they are planning to do. When they receive assistance, support, love and interest (and medical treatment if necessary) the majority can be dissuaded from suicide.

This is particularly true of adolescents. After the difficult years they move on; they build new lives.

The most insidiously evil myth of all is that nothing can be done to stop young people committing suicide.

YOUTH SUICIDE: THE FACTS

More young Australians are dying from suicide and motor vehicle accidents than from any other cause.

In 1995, according to the Australian Bureau of Statistics (ABS), suicide was the recorded cause of death of 350 young men and 84 young women – a total of 434 people aged fifteen to twenty-four. Motor vehicle accidents killed 594 young people.

Because of the government's wide ranging commitment to reducing the road toll, deaths from motor vehicle accidents are decreasing. Deaths from suicide are not.

For each completed suicide, at least thirty, and probably more than forty, other young people attempt to take their lives. These figures are unconfirmed conservative estimates as there is no accurate reporting system applied to cases of attempted suicide.

While young men are four times more likely to complete the act of suicide than young women, females are more likely than the males to attempt to take their own lives.

According to the ABS the number of young Australian males (15–24) committing suicide increased by almost fifty percent over the fifteen years between 1979 and 1993 and peaked in 1988.

It's possible that more males die by suicide than females mainly because of the methods they use. Young men generally choose violent means of death, such as shooting, hanging, jumping from bridges or cliffs or throwing themselves in front of trains – acts which kill them instantly. Young women tend to choose poisoning through the ingestion of tablets or gas and are therefore more likely to be saved through medical intervention.

Over recent years, the standardised death rate for suicide has remained relatively stable in Australia, ranging from 2,161 in 1990 to 2,367 in 1995. However, this stability obscures considerable increases in particular age and sex groups – specifically, the increase in the number of youth suicides as well as an even greater increase in suicides by men aged twenty-five to forty-four.

Young people most at risk of suicide in this country include young Aboriginal men and young men living in rural areas.

Rates of suicide represent the actual number of suicides expressed as a proportion of every 100,000 people in a specific age and sex group. The rate of suicide among young males of Aboriginal and Torres Strait Islander descent is believed to be more than double that of the overall population, at around 70 per 100,000 (Queensland Health, 1990–2).

As we saw in *Country kids: who cares?*, young men living in rural and remote areas have a consistently higher rate of suicide than those in urban areas. The rate of suicide among young males in rural areas has increased more than fifty percent since 1986, from 24 deaths per 100,000 population in that year to 37 in 1992. This is a thirty-three percent increase in the number of deaths among young urban males for the same period (24 per 100,000).

The increase in rural deaths is probably connected with the devastation caused by drought, the economic downturn in country towns and by access to guns. Over fifty percent of rural male suicides use guns, compared with twenty-three percent among urban males.

The incidence of suicide rises with age during adolescence, so it is rare below the age of twelve but increases rapidly through the teen years and into the early twenties. The highest rate of suicide in Australia occurs in men aged twenty-five to forty-four. Some health professionals believe that many of these men attempted or at least contemplated suicide in their earlier years, that the seeds of their depression were sown during that time and that the opportunity to prevent subsequent tragic loss of life was lost through lack of effective intervention during adolescence.

When writing on youth suicide, it is difficult to settle on accurate statistics. The criteria for reporting suicide and attempted suicide vary from state to state and protocols are not standardised even among hospitals in the same cities. Almost certainly the figures for both attempted and completed suicide are actually much higher than the ones given here. While deaths which have not resulted from natural causes have to be reported to the coroner, state coroners are frequently limited by lack of clear evidence in their ability to make a finding of death by suicide. Self-inflicted injuries are widely under-reported by hospitals; deaths from drug overdoses and 'accidental' poisoning may be suicides.

While young people have been dying in motor vehicle accidents for many years, most researchers now believe that deaths by suicide in the fifteen to twenty-four year age group now come close to outnumbering the deaths of young people on the roads. Unexplained single vehicle accidents could well be suicides, but in the absence of conclusive evidence the coroner is bound to bring down a verdict of accidental death, a pronouncement to which few bereaved families object.

In 1995, across all age groups, more Australians died by suicide than on the roads. There were 2,367 suicides, while 2029 were killed in motor vehicle accidents. However, in the fifteen to twenty-four year age group, in the three years from 1993 to 1995, the number of deaths from motor vehicle traffic accidents exceeded the number of reported deaths from suicide in this age group.

Data concerning attempted suicide is even more unreliable, being limited to hospital reports of people treated for self-harming behaviour and self-inflicted injuries. Researchers believe that the official rates for attempted suicide could be underestimated by sixty to seventy percent. However, hospital figures clearly indicate that the rate of self-inflicted injury for both males and females peaks in the fifteen to twenty-four age group. Once again, such injuries include drug overdoses, poisoning by alcohol, tablets or gas, and razor or knife wounds.

COMPARISONS WITH OTHER COUNTRIES

At 26.6 deaths per 100,000 of population in 1990–91, the suicide rate in Australia for males in the fifteen to twenty-four age group was the fourth highest among fourteen countries in the industrialised world. According to statistics prepared by the World Health Organization, only New Zealand, Canada and Norway have higher rates. The rate for young females dying by suicide is much lower, at 6.2, but this is still the fourth highest rate in the industrialised world, ranking us behind New Zealand, Norway and Switzerland.

Spain and Italy have particularly low rates of youth suicide, particularly among young men. What do these nations have that we in the so-called lucky country have missed? What are they doing that the people in our wide brown land, with its turquoise oceans and its democracy and its mateship … are not?

CAUSES

Mental health problems, particularly depression, have been identified as the main risk factors for suicide in young people. In more basic terms, many of our young people are so unhappy that they have become ill. Their depression stems from many things including physical and sexual abuse, family conflict, drug abuse, unemployment, confusion about their sexuality and gender, emotional neglect, pressure to perform, and hopelessness. There is also evidence that genetic factors may affect depressive illness.

Friends, relatives and hospital records indicate that about ninety percent of the young people who die by suicide had indication of mental illness – in many cases, depression.

Probably eighty percent warn their nearest and dearest in some way and forty to fifty percent go to a GP and report minor health problems (that is, not mental health) in the month preceding the suicide. Very few young people who kill themselves are receiving psychiatric treatment for a recognised illness.

Little is known about Aboriginal youth suicide, the effects of irresponsible media reports that sensationalise suicide (and which are alleged by some psychiatrists to cause copy-cat deaths), why youth suicide sometimes occurs in clusters, rural youth suicide and the effects of long-term unemployment on the suicide rate.

Quite a lot of information about the connection between illicit drugs and suicide is now available – particularly the depressive effects of prolonged marijuana use on the human brain; too many informed people, for reasons of their own, are preferring to ignore this information, rather than trade it for the lives and futures of our young people.

Despite the increasing incidence of suicide and growing concern both in the government and in the community, no accurate record of how many people complete suicide in Australia exists. All that we know for certain is that young people access medical services very little, young men least of all and young men in rural areas hardly ever.

Youth suicide in Australia — the facts

- In 1995, 434 young men and women aged 15–24 committed suicide. Of these, 350 were males.
- For every one of these deaths, at least forty other young people attempted to commit suicide.
- The suicide rate for young men is far higher than that of young women, although this is partly balanced by a higher rate of attempted suicide among young women.
- The rate of suicide for young men in Australia increased by 50% between 1979 and 1993. This has been consistent with an increased rate for men aged 25–44 for the same period.
- The male suicide rate among rural young men is higher than the rate for urban young men and is increasing.
- The suicide rate for Aboriginal men aged 15–29 is at least double that of other young people, including rural youth, and has been increasing since the 1980s.
- More young people die from suicide and motor vehicle accidents than from any other cause.
- The suicide rate of young men is relatively high in Australia compared with other countries, but is not the highest.
- The main contributing factors are depression and loss of hope.

Compiled with the assistance of David de Vaus,
Australian Institute of Family Studies.

TO THE WORLD

Alone I am as I sit at the lake's edge throwing pebbles.
The colour of my soul is so black, my heart so heavy,
That even the pleasant sound of robins drifting from a
  nearby glade
Cannot soothe my feelings of bitterness and emptiness.

The warmth of the sun does not reach me
as I hide behind a face of questionable character.
Who is this person who is always gay and nonchalant?
A second self perhaps ... a creature born out of a search for
  sanctuary
Simply a lifeless carcass to hide within during times of display.

Trust, faithfulness, compassion ... words which no longer
  hold meaning for me,
Have been replaced with betrayal, isolation and
  worthlessness,
All blended together to create this dark and sour being which
  is my true self.

I long for the day when I can feel love, happiness and a sense
  of purpose again.
Surely there will come a time when the seed of life
Which has been planted and buried deep inside of me
Can blossom into something wonderful, something special,
  something joyous to behold.
Please nourish me ... Let me grow ... I yearn to live ...
                                    Adam Kemp, October 1995

This poem was written three months before Adam Kemp
took his life in January 1996, at the age of nineteen.

PART TWO

COLLIN: CARS, CARES, CATASTROPHES

JAN: 'Three months after he began his apprenticeship with Repco, Collin had a terrible car accident. He had joined a group of boys who bought old motorbikes and even older cars and did them up. Collin had sold his motorbike to buy an old Holden although he was still only on his L-plates; he wasn't old enough to get his licence.

'At the time of the accident he was driving his car with a friend in the passenger seat. He had concussion, broken ribs, a broken knee, black eyes. His mate rang us at 11 p.m. and Ron and I raced to the hospital. He was a long time mending and for years afterwards he had trouble with his leg. It didn't cure him of cars. As the accident was not his fault, he was never charged and he did not accept that he been doing anything wrong.

'Collin could never comprehend that rules – any rules – applied to him as well as to everyone else. But despite this attitude to authority, he was still such a nice kid. The number of fights he had with us could be counted on one hand. He was lovely to his sisters, he was great with his little brother and kind and considerate with me. He adored his grandmother. When he heard she had had a heart attack, he beat me to the hospital and arrived in tears ... and how he didn't get a speeding ticket *that* day I'll never know!

'But he began distancing himself from Ron. We would lie awake for hours, talking about our growing concern for him. We were worried that he would die in a car. The cars he was working on were becoming more and more powerful.

'Cathy had left school after getting a brilliant pass in the Higher School Certificate. She was studying biomedical science at the University of Technology in Sydney. Julianne was doing very well at school. Adam, like Collin, was more of a plodder. I returned to part-time work at a child care centre when Adam was five and remained there for five years, until I joined the accounts staff at the local council.

'Collin had a beautiful personality; people of all ages were attracted to him. But he distrusted people in authority. He particularly hated the police. In fact we had to tell him not to discuss his feelings in front of Julianne and Adam as we didn't want them growing up thinking they couldn't trust policemen.

'He was booked for speeding so many times that he lost his provisional licence. We made him sell his car.

'We could still do that – insist on him selling the car. We have brought up our kids to be obedient. If Mum and Dad say "no", it means "no". Their friends would say: "Just go and ask them again" and they would say: "Why? No means no."

'I used to think it was good but now I believe that's a terrible thing we did to them. I'm not proud of it. Why did they think they couldn't ask us to change our minds? Why did they never stand up to us?

'I was brought up to believe that if you put everybody else first and you set yourself last and you would be a good person. That's what I taught Cathy and Collin to do. And even now what I absolutely love best about every one of my children is that they are nice people. They were nice kids and they are nice young adults. Collin was a worry but he was good to other people.

'As a teenager Collin had lots of girlfriends but when he was eighteen he became seriously involved with Sharon. It was a love-hate relationship. They fought all the time. They were on and off, on and off. Her family were volatile – having rows and making up again was quite normal. Collin spent a lot of time with them and got on well with them. They really liked him. We liked Sharon too, although we didn't like all the fighting. We welcomed her into our family. I made clothes for her, she slept here frequently – although not with him. That's something I could never condone, not under our roof. Not even now. It goes too deep. Perhaps it's hypocritical, knowing they are having sex yet not allowing it at home. But we couldn't.

'Collin moved out at nineteen and lived in our old renovated shack with a few mates but that didn't work out. He came home after about six months because he wasn't happy there. Material things were important to Collin. He liked living in a nice house. He and his mates had cleaned up the shack before he moved in, and he wouldn't let Sharon smoke inside. But I think he preferred living at home.

'They moved into a place together when he was twenty-one. By that time Collin had finished his apprenticeship. He failed the technical college course but the company kept him on anyway. They don't usually do that but he had formidable mechanical skills. Sharon worked in an office. Collin continued to spend most of his time working on cars. He had quite a nice settlement from the car accident and he bought a speed boat, so they used to spend a lot of time on that as well.

'They had a dog, a bull terrier named Munro after Munro Shock Absorbers. Collin told us this hilarious story about the day when they were all up at the dam and he and his friends were throwing sticks into the water for Munro to go and fetch. Somebody threw a rock into the dam and Munro went after that as well. It was a very large rock and Munro was too stupid to let go. They waited and waited but Munro didn't come up. Collin had to dive into the dam and save the dog; he pulled him out and gave him the kiss of life. Munro looked better after it than Collin did.

'Then Collin was in another car accident. He had internal bleeding, a brain haemorrhage and he broke his other leg. We should have got counselling for him after that. We didn't think about it, but it might have helped.

'Collin had always put on a front of absolutely loathing all drugs. When I asked him why he no longer saw certain friends he would say to me: "Mum, you think they are nice but they are the biggest potheads around". I had no idea he was smoking marijuana. I can remember times when he was absolutely paranoid with fear and worry, convinced that the police and the dog squad were after him and that he would be locked up. I was too naive to realise it was probably drugs that made him that way. I put it down to genuine fear and the drink. I knew he started drinking from the age of about twenty. He never drank beer; he drank heavier stuff like Southern Comfort. We never tried to stop him from drinking. Our friends drink. We are a bit unusual because we don't, but that doesn't mean we expect others not to.

'When Collin was in his early twenties I became seriously concerned about what was making him unhappy and Ron and I raised the subject of suicide with him. Three mates in a large crowd to which Collin belonged had killed themselves in the previous couple of years. We only knew one of them personally and although Ron and I went to the funeral, Collin didn't. When we asked him why, he said he couldn't face it.

'We sat down with him then and said all the wrong things. I said what a terrible thing to do to the family. All the advice we offered was based on looking at what tragedy is left behind. What we have learned since of course, is that suicidal people are in no fit state to think of what is left behind; they don't give a damn. They just want to get out.

'One afternoon in September 1991, Collin left his flat, left Sharon, quit his job, got in his car and drove to Queensland.

'At first we didn't know where he was, but he rang after a couple of days. I talked to him for hours on the phone and I sort of planted the idea of going to stay with his aunt, Ron's sister-in-law, who lives up north with her husband and sons; I prayed that he would stay there for a while and get a job. I didn't want him coming back to whatever demons were waiting for him here.

'He wouldn't let us tell Sharon where he was. Six weeks later he came home, saying he missed her, that he couldn't be without her. We had just moved into this house and he came back to live with us. His relationship with Sharon continued to disintegrate. He seemed very unhappy to me.

'One day I said to him: "Collin, what exactly is the *matter* with you?" I remember his face so clearly when he replied. He was very handsome, with long dark curly hair which was the fashion at the time. "Mum," he said, "I'm just so angry all the time inside".

'I knew then that we were all in trouble. I knew that his anger was our fault because we had forced him to bottle it up inside; we had taught him it wasn't "nice" to fight.

'I asked Collin if he would talk about his feelings to a counsellor and to my surprise he agreed. I found someone at a private clinic and paid for Collin to go. I didn't know you could get counselling at public hospitals without paying huge fees. But I felt better that Collin was getting help. He went five or six times.

'Collin lived at home with us for about three months and then there was some sort of altercation about his driving; a policeman came to the door and said there had been a complaint. But when Collin said he would move out, it came from out of the blue really.

'So he went. He stayed away for about four months. He lived in a house with his mate, Jaakko, and his girlfriend, Lindy. I continued to worry about him, with good reason as it turned out. One day I ran into Sharon's mother in the street and she said she was very worried about Collin. It made me wonder if she knew something I didn't. I came home and told Ron to go and tell Collin we wanted him back. When he came home to us we made no conditions. We loved him. I thought at twenty-two he was old enough to be permitted to live the way he wanted to.

'The following six months were the happiest we had had for many years. Our daughter, Cathy, had been badly hurt by the break-up of a long relationship with a young pilot, but then she met Dean* and they became engaged. The whole family was involved in the wedding plans.

'The only obvious problem Collin had at that time was that he and Sharon were still having trouble getting on. I finally said to him: "Collin, I just can't go on like this with you and Sharon any more. I have the other kids to think about. One minute you love her, the next minute you're telling them to say you're not here when you are. I don't want Sharon coming here or ringing up until you two have sorted things out between you". For two months we didn't see or hear from her.

'There was an incident during that time – Collin started going out with a girl he really liked but then he was warned that her boyfriend was in gaol and could be dangerous when he got out. Collin came home worried to the point of tears.

'Then Sharon came back.

'We were all getting ready for the wedding by then and she wanted to join in the excitement. Collin's car was to be the wedding car and he was going to drive Cathy to the church.

'His mind must have been in turmoil. Everything was revolving around the wedding and he was playing an important part in it. What we didn't know was that he had lost his licence again. I had my suspicions, but I decided to say nothing.

'The car Collin was driving at the time, the one that was to carry the bride, was an HR Holden which he had spent years doing up. It would have been worth a lot of money to people who were interested. It was his life – his whole self-esteem seemed to be dependent on that car.

'I love old cars myself. It was beautiful and it was well looked after. It was bright and shiny and everyone noticed it. But it cost a lot of money to run and it was so finely tuned that it often broke down. And let's face it, the police target those sort of vehicles. "Get rid of it, Collin," I used to tell him. "It's causing you so much pain." I can't believe that I actually told him that car was a noose around his neck.

'And then, finally, I discovered what may have been at the root of Collin's problems. Six months earlier he had apparently hit a man at some club. He had told me about it – Collin was never aggressive and I believed him when he said the other fellow and his mate had been following him and abusing him, although Collin had definitely thrown the first punch.

'However, the fellow had belatedly put in a complaint to the police. When I read the statement which Collin had signed, it was a very different story to the one he had given me.

'"This isn't right," I said to him. "Why did you sign it? Didn't you read it first?"

'After a pause he said the police had asked him to read his statement aloud to them, to verify that it was correct. "It was taking me so long," he said, "...to read it out. So they just said sign it and I did."

'I had known he wasn't a good reader. But I had no idea he couldn't read something as simple as this, that he couldn't pick up obvious differences in what the words meant.

'Later I discovered from his counsellor that Collin was illiterate.

'This was why he hated school. It was why he had been behind in ten English assignments – as late as it was, why wasn't it picked up then? It was why he played up in school. It was why he couldn't even pass the tech course. He couldn't read the words on the charge sheets. My son couldn't *read*.

'He had become very clever over the years at covering this up. He appeared to read car magazines from cover to cover. I think maybe he could understand language relating to car parts.

'I thought he did badly at school because he didn't study. As it turns out, he may have been trying very hard, but he gave up because it was just too hard. He could understand maths and science, but English and reading and writing were beyond him.

'It was because of this that he was convinced he was a failure.'

RON: 'Cars were his life. At one stage he had three – an FJ ute, an HR Holden and a Statesman. Collin never had much money; he did them up by bartering for parts. His social life was non-existent. He'd work on his cars and his friends' cars twenty-four hours a day if he could; he couldn't help himself.

'He found himself a girlfriend who was willing to sit in the gutter smoking cigarettes and watching him work on cars, day after day. She spat the dummy occasionally but she always came back. Time after time he'd say he was never going to see her again. He didn't take her out. He didn't even see her to the door when she left our house.

'I believe Collin loved Sharon in his own way. I also know he wanted to get out of the relationship on many occasions.

'Collin hated authority. His attitude to the police was intolerable in a home like ours. But kids are influenced by so many things other than families these days. They see reports on the media, they watch violence on television and movies. They spend much more time with their peers than they used to do. Parents now have a much smaller role in the destiny of their children.

'Collin hated rules. He wanted to be free. He was brainwashed into thinking that was the way life should be. He was a revhead and he hung around with revheads. All they wanted to do was drink and race around in their hotted-up cars. He would come and watch a violent movie on his own rather than watch a family movie with the rest of us.

'You can imagine how the police around here reacted to Collin's cars. They pulled him up and served defect notices on him every chance they found. But Collin was a tearaway. He would chuck a wheelie right in front of a police car. He would purposely provoke them.

'I'd say: "Why don't you get a car they won't notice?" He would reply: "Haven't I got the right to drive any car I want?" I told him that sometimes in life we have to do as we are told, but that didn't sit well with Collin.

'One night, after a bad car accident, in which he broke his leg, he was parked with Sharon on the airstrip out in the bush. The police drove up and shone their headlights on them. So Collin put his lights on high beam and shone them at the police. They ordered him out of the car but when he reached into the back for his crutches they pulled a gun on him and radioed for assistance. They thought he had a rifle in the back seat.

'We don't live far from the airstrip. Cars went screaming past our house and we wondered what was going on. They searched him, grabbed his wallet and threw all his personal cards on the ground.

'It was his fault initially, but they did harass him. Collin's counsellor rang them once to ask them why. He explained that Collin was having some problems. The police told him they'd get him any way they could.

'I thought: "The wheel always turns. Everyone goes a bit wild when they are young. Then they settle down. That's what happens in life".

'One day I heard an excruciating scream of wheels spinning that just went on and on. A massive great ball of white smoke rose up above the trees to what seemed like one hundred feet in the air. After a while Collin appeared in his HR – now driving at ten kilometres an hour because the road outside our house could damage his delicate suspension!

'A local policeman soon arrived at the door. "This sort of thing just has to stop," he told me. "I like Collin. I know he is a nice kid. Just tell him to behave."

'I had a terrible row with Collin that afternoon. We are not a family who has trouble with the police. I told Collin if he lived in my house he had to live within the law. He wouldn't see reason. He packed up and moved out that night. Jan was very unhappy about it. But it was Collin's decision to go.

'He lived in a rented house with a mate for six months. It was one of the few times in his adult life when he wasn't working, but he never asked us for money and he was too proud to go on the dole. He was drinking. Apparently he was also using some drugs.

'Jan went down in secret to have a cup of tea with him and offer him money. She hoped he would come home for Mothers' Day but he didn't, because he had no money to buy her a present.

'I learned much later – too much later – that he attempted to take his own life twice during that time. The first time he tried to slash his wrists but a friend stayed with him all night, talking him out of it. The second time he tried to gas himself in the car. Typically, he ran out of petrol.

'I believe I actually saw Collin the day after that second attempt. I had asked him to look at a new car I was going to buy. He drove it very slowly and he was so sick he could hardly get his head under the bonnet. I didn't know what was wrong with him.

'If only their mates knew that by telling people what is happening they have a better chance of preventing it happening again.

'I couldn't understand his attitude. I had taught him to take the good times and laugh. But when the bad times come you don't just roll over and play dead. On the subject of suicide I had said it was a cowardly act and I would never forgive anyone who did that to their family.

'Finally Jan got really worried about him so I went and brought him home. We then had a really good six months, although he lost his licence again during that time. He didn't tell us. He knew if he did I wouldn't let him drive the wedding car.

'Then one Friday afternoon he came into the house and showed me a petrol cap. "Look at this, Dad," he said. "This is the start of my next car."

'He went off to his room in a really good mood, but then he found two letters on his table. We learned later that the first letter said he was free to apply for a new licence. The other was a fine for driving without a licence, which meant he wouldn't get his licence back after all, or at least, not in time for the wedding. He came out and asked Julianne if she had left his mail in there. She said she hadn't.

'"Shit," he said to her. "It must have been Mum." He assumed, rightly, that Jan would have guessed what was in the letters.

'Then he went down to our shed, which I have set up as a bit of a gym. I could hear him banging about in there for a long time. He seemed to be belting the stuffing out of the punching bag. I didn't know what he was angry about.

'Not long afterwards Sharon came to pick him up and they went out. He called: "See ya, Dad" and I waved.'

CATHY: 'Collin did speed in his car, of course he did. But the police targeted him more than the others. They used to sit outside his work and follow him home. If he went even a little over the speed limit they would fine him. He used to get so frustrated but there was nothing he could do about it. So instead of just copping the fine, he would give them lip. Then they'd book him for something else so he would give them more. And so it went on.

'He started building an image for himself. He wore black jeans, leather boots, a leather vest with tassels hanging off it. He liked looking tough. Collin and his friends looked like bad guys but they weren't really. All they were interested in was cars.

'We didn't have a lot to do with each other once we grew up. I was away at university; I was always studying and trying to find time to see my boyfriend. Funnily enough, I did better with Collin when I talked to him on the phone. I knew he was very depressed and sometimes he'd ring me and talk about his friends who had committed suicide. I said to him: "If it ever gets that bad, ring me, even if it's four in the morning". He never said he was going to do it but he talked about it in a way that indicated to me that he thought it might not be such a bad solution.

'I could see why he was depressed. He had cast himself into this mould and it wasn't really him but he couldn't change it. I think it's a pretty shitty world myself but for Collin it was worse. It was getting reinforced to him all the time that there was nothing fair in life.

'Life was hard work for Collin. All the things that should have given him pleasure didn't. The family didn't. Sharon didn't. In the end all his self-esteem was centred on his car. So if anything happened to the car – and things were always happening to it – it was a major blow.

'A lady crashed into it once and she got out and she said: "Oh, thank goodness it's only an old Holden". And it *wasn't* an old Holden. It was a beautiful car and he had poured so much time and effort and money into it. It had to be looking good, it had to be running well and if it wasn't he would stew and stew. There was always a problem getting the money to repair it.

'His friends hurt him. When he moved into our old shack with some mates and they didn't look after it he was furious. He had a lot of friends but he told me people only ever hung out with him so he would fix their cars.

'Then there was his relationship with Sharon which was just so difficult. It was always him breaking it off, never her. She loved Collin with everything she had; no other girl was allowed to look at him. She couldn't live without him, but she gave a lot in return. Mum brought us up all equal – we can all cook and wash and clean. But Sharon would do everything for Collin. I think sometimes it was just too intense for him. He preferred to split up rather than have a screaming match.

'Collin told me he couldn't read or write but I didn't believe him. I knew he had been to school. I said: "Of *course* you can read, Collin". I mean, how could he have read the assembly instructions when he was working on engines? I thought he meant: "I can't read as well as you".

'Once when I went home Collin reached his arm across in front of me and just beneath the cuff of his sleeve, I saw a huge scar. I was horrified. I grabbed his hand and said: "What *have* you done to yourself? It looks as though you've slashed your wrist." He said he had burnt it on the exhaust pipe. Sharon backed him up. My mind wouldn't let me believe what he might have been trying to do and I let it go.

'Collin kept us at a distance – the exception was Julianne. She hugged him all the time.

'I broke up with my boyfriend, Trevor, in 1991, after seven years, and then I met Dean and we decided to get married a year later. There was a bit of trouble about the wedding.

Mum wanted Collin to wear nice clothes when he was driving us to the church. He wanted to wear his black gear and his leather vest with the tassels. He didn't want to wear what to him were poofy clothes. He said that wasn't who he was. But just a week before the wedding I was home and he seemed fine. As Dean and I were backing out in the car, Collin was striding down the yard yelling out at Sharon: "Of *course* I'm gonna get a haircut!" And I drove home thinking: "Great. He has sorted himself out. I don't have to worry about him".'

JULIANNE: 'There was a big gap between Cathy and me and Adam was only little. Collin and I were the middle kids. When he started working on cars I used to go downstairs to his room and talk to him, the same as I did when he was little and doing the bikes.

'He went off to do his own thing a lot as he got older, but he wasn't as independent as you'd think; he wasn't emotionally strong. Dad has this amazing willpower but Collin was the sort to go along with the crowd.

'When he went to live with his friend Jaakko he took me into his room one day and picked up a sheaf of papers. "Look at this," he said. "These are all fines, all fines and I can't pay them".

'I used to talk to him for hours about girls and cars and his friends and Sharon. That was about the full range of subjects you could talk to him about. He wasn't very philosophical. As he got older, he'd say: "Life sucks and then you die". I remember thinking it wasn't a good thing to be saying, but you know – when you're sixteen and your brother's your hero, you can't imagine anything being all that wrong.'

SHARON is tall, blonde and tanned; beautiful without a trace of make-up, she could have stepped straight out of 'Baywatch' – a gorgeous Australian sheila on a golden stretch of sand. In reality, both her parents are English, and she is more comfortable making tea in her kitchen than hanging around the beach. Sharon is now twenty-six years old and six months pregnant with her second child.

She speaks quietly about her years with Collin Schultz, but she is subdued – she has a new partner now and she makes it clear that her top priority is her two-year-old son. Sharon is the first to acknowledge that motherhood has softened the sharper edges of her personality; the new role has not, however, persuaded her to give up cigarettes.

'You could talk about anything to Collin, but mostly it was cars. He didn't play any team sports or anything like that. He was a mad car freak and I got interested in cars because of him.

'We met when we were in Year Ten and we were good friends at first because he was so easy-going and nice. We started going together when we were seventeen, after we had left school. He had just had this big car accident and I went to see him at the hospital every day. I liked him so much. He was gorgeous looking and he had a kind heart. There was so much about him that was great. I thought he was a pretty bright person, too.

'I helped him build the HR Holden. We went through two shells – he stripped them for parts. I had an HR too; I bought it from the wreckers when it had a big ding in the back. Collin did it up for me and we sprayed it; it looked great after that. It was my first car.

'We broke up a lot because he had the old roving eye; he always came back to me. He was friendly to everyone, but he couldn't show his deeper emotions the way I would have liked him to do. I tried to get him to talk about the problems he had with his family but he'd only do it every now and then.

'He felt he was the rebel of the family. He couldn't communicate at all with them, although I got on well with them myself. The contrast between Collin's family and mine was incredible. We all love each other a lot but we have slanging matches all the time. You *never* argued at the Schultz's.

'Collin and I had a good time together. We went to the sailing club sometimes and when Collin got the speed boat we went water-skiing a lot. Of course, we went to heaps of car shows.

'Then he had his second accident. He was the passenger. We had this joke in our crowd – if you were in an accident and Collin was in the car, he'd be sure to come out of it worse than you. He had a big pin put in his leg, but he never whinged about his injuries. You never knew if the accidents affected him.

'Collin wasn't really a drinker. He got so sick at his eighteenth birthday party he didn't touch alcohol for about two years. He didn't socialise much. He would drop me at the club to be with my friends and go home to work on his car. He didn't like dancing.

'Sometimes when we broke up he saw other girls. After I met Collin I only ever went out with someone else once, but he didn't like it. I was very loyal to him.

'When we were in our early twenties Collin started getting very depressed. He never had enough money to do what he wanted with the cars. He wanted things that were out of his reach. Once he got real fed up and ran away to Queensland. I probably should have resolved never to have anything more to do with him after that, because I felt so hurt, but I couldn't. I loved him too much.

'It was when he was living with a mate that he tried to kill himself the first time. We had been to a rock concert and he went home with a bottle of Southern Comfort and Coke. He rang me a few hours later. He said: "Shaz, can you come over, I'm not feeling real well".

'When I got there he was sitting on the floor beside the phone. He said to me: "I ran out of petrol". I went into the garage and realised he had tried to gas himself. I saw the hose sticking out of the exhaust pipe. I tried to tell him everything would be all right but he said he was fed up with life. I told him he had to think of his parents. I told him he had to think of me.

'There had to be something wrong with Collin for him to do that. I mean, I did the same things Collin did. I drank. I smoked a bit of dope. The last thing I would ever do is kill myself. My grandmother used to tell us about the War and the Depression. It makes you wonder what any of us have to whinge about.

'He started seeing a counsellor, but he didn't want his friends to know. I don't know why because his mates were nice people. They would not have minded. I just hoped he would say something about it all to the counsellor, because those people would know what to do.

'Collin's personality didn't go well with alcohol. It bought out lots of aggro in him. He wasn't permanently depressed. He didn't drink every night of the week but when he did, when he was down or worried, he would go on a binge. I don't think his mother had any idea.

'Normally Collin was such a beautiful person. Everyone he spoke to loved him.

'His parents didn't mind him being into the cars and doing them up, but they didn't like him getting into trouble with the police the way he did. I'd have been the same if I was them. I'd be scared of what might happen to my son if he was in strife with the law.

'I could have understood why he was so depressed if he had been in really deep trouble, if he was a bad guy, if he was behaving like a complete arsehole all the time. But he wasn't. He was just Collin and I loved him very much.'

'HOW CAN YOU TELL IF A KID'S GOING TO . . . ?'

Most suicidal young people don't actually want to die. They just want to stop living long enough to escape from their pain.

Suicidal people have tunnel vision. They are in the depths of despair and they simply cannot see any other way of solving their problems. They are swimming against a tide of depression, and it may only take one more small wave to push them into waters so deep and unfathomable that they feel they are drowning. Death offers itself as an alternative to the struggle to stay afloat.

'It's a conscious decision but that doesn't mean it's a rational decision,' said Victorian youth suicide prevention specialist, Barry Taylor. 'They don't understand the consequences of their action; they don't understand the finality of death.

'Young people don't have very good internal monitoring systems. Often they don't even realise how bad they are feeling.

'A young girl goes home and takes some pills. A young man gets into his car and drives straight into a truck on the highway. Somebody finds the girl before the pills take effect. Nobody can save the boy. One dies, one doesn't. At least not this time. Whether the girl tries again will depend on how much help she gets.

'If we teach them life skills from an early age and give them help when they need it, they could get over these crises and after a short period of trauma, they can go on with their lives. They may never need help again.'

'When that moment of choice arrives, they are wearing blinkers,' said Margaret Appleby, the founder of the Rose Foundation, an organisation working towards suicide prevention. 'Survivors say that when they became suicidal they could only see blackness ahead, not even a trace of grey. In a way that's reassuring for their families – that it wasn't lack of love, it was just total despair'.

Suicidal people feel as if they are failures. They see their future as being very bleak and they feel powerless to change their life. They don't have the energy. They see no other way to go. They have no hope.

Many of them go to a doctor and without mentioning they are considering taking their lives, give veiled clues about their state of mind.

Some young suicidal people actually seem to believe they will be around to see the effects of their death on the people they love. Rational thinking is suspended; they think that in some way they will be able to witness the consequences of their actions. The younger they are the more likely they are to act impulsively. If there has been a catalyst such as a hard school exam, or a broken romance, they may actually imagine they will see how their teacher/parents/girlfriend or boyfriend will suffer when she or he discovers they are dead. Presumably, somewhere on the other side of their troubled imagination, all will then be forgiven and life will resume.

In one breath they threaten to kill themselves in the afternoon and in the next they worry aloud about how much study they need to do before next Friday's exam. A young woman who made a tape for her parents before she took her life spoke of her marriage and career plans and her excitement at the thought of travelling in the years ahead.

'What I can't handle at the moment though' she admitted, 'is my immediate future.'

Suicide victims are on a see-saw which dips them low into a hollow of hopelessness, then swings them up into the reality of routine. Confronting them with their plans for death – asking them outright if that's what they might do – may be the only way to bring their lives back into balance.

SUICIDE SIGNALS

The most important sign that a young person is contemplating taking their own life is when they talk, write, hint or even draw pictures about death.

A morbid preoccupation with the subject of death or means of dying should never be ignored.

A girl from one school noticed that a boy in her class always filled the blank spaces on his study sheets with doodles of a noose hanging over a half-open door. After several months, she noticed that the noose in one of these doodles was no longer empty – the boy had drawn a body hanging from the rope. She took the picture to the school counsellor who was already seeing the boy. The counsellor had been afraid to ask him if he felt suicidal. His parents were contacted and when confronted, the boy admitted he was planning to kill himself during the coming weekend.

Hints, such as: 'Nobody would care if I wasn't here', should not be ignored or trivialised. It's very easy to do – the busy mother, rushing to get the washing on the line before work – is incredulous that on top of everything else she has on her overflowing plate she is expected to ladle out some sympathy for a self-pitying adolescent. But she needs to know more. She needs to ask and to listen.

Jason Connor, talking to his best mate on his mobile, said he was going away for a while. 'Ring us when you get there,' exhorted his friend. 'Mate,' said Jason, 'where I'm going, I don't think there'll be a phone.'

A second and more obvious sign that a young person is suicidal is depression. This is less likely to be laughed off or joked about by the family – a constantly miserable adolescent is never a joking matter. Long-faced and lethargic, they often lie around like a piece of the lounge suite – and they are just as hard to move. Alternately, they may be angry and uncooperative all the time.

Depressed young people, like anyone else suffering from a depressed state of mind, need help, whether it's medical help or simply someone to whom they can talk. (Sadly, they may not *want* to talk to anyone.)

An absolutely critical indication that a young person is thinking about committing suicide is a sudden burst of cheerfulness. According to suicide prevention educators, more people die as a result of an apparent improvement than at any other time.

They have been feeling gloomy and down, they haven't been sleeping, they've lost weight, they've been worrying everyone around them – and suddenly, for no obvious reason, they cheer up. They throw off their depression, they laugh, they talk, they appear to be at peace.

All too often the improvement is a result of the fact that the young person concerned has made a decision to stop living and in the relief of this decision, their problems no longer concern them.

Whatever happens to Mum and Dad, it's no longer going to be their concern. Who cares if their girlfriend or boyfriend starts seeing someone else? They won't be around to watch. The possibility that they may be homosexual, learning to speak English properly, what they look like, whether their skin clears up, how much weight they've lost or gained, how smart they are, coping with the Shakespeare project, understanding physics, being loved – none of this will matter if they're dead. They don't have to study; he won't ever have to look in the employment section of the paper again. After tomorrow she won't have to lie in her darkened bedroom, teeth and knees clenched together, watching fearfully for the door to silently open.

After months of depression, during which she wouldn't or couldn't do her school work, a sixteen-year-old girl from a country town told her parents she was turning over a new leaf. 'I've got a major assignment due; I want to study. I want to really make you all proud of me.' Her parents were delighted and left her to her work. They arrived home from the shops to find her hanging from a tree in the garden.

If the circumstances of the person are unchanged, if nothing has happened to lift the young person out of their stupor of misery, there is a strong possibility that the only thing that is cheering them up is that they have found a way to escape from their problems.

A woman with three teenage sons remembers the night before one of them died as being the happiest evening the family had shared for months. 'For once he came out and joined us in front of the television and we all spent the night together – it was lovely.'

If hopeless and helpless feelings go on for too long without intervention, adolescents can get sucked down into the muddy depths of despair, unable to pull themselves out of the bog.

With hindsight, families remember signs that their children may not have been coping, but it's often difficult to detect unusual behaviour when you see a person every day, when life is rushed and busy and there's never enough time to finish the ironing, let alone smooth the creases from everyone's psyches.

People contemplating suicide often withdraw from their families and their friends because of their guilt or anger. They feel so badly about themselves that they believe their presence must be a burden to those they love. They become very quiet and spend a long time in their rooms or in solitary places.

Adam Kemp's mother said he spent hours in his bedroom, playing his music and using his computer. She thought it was a typical teenage thing; she felt it would be wrong to invade his privacy by going in there to talk to him; she hoped he would come out when he was ready. If by some miracle her son was back in his room today, she says, she would not wait to be invited in.

Teachers may be more likely to notice serious changes in a young person's demeanour and attitude, mainly because they are used to measuring behavioural norms. If a quiet and shy person suddenly becomes very loud and brazen, or the reverse occurs – if a student is repeatedly getting into trouble – it's a classroom clue that all may not be right.

Another very obvious sign that a young person is considering taking his or her own life is an attempt to put their affairs in order. Many of them give away their possessions, even things they have always treasured. They distribute their favourite CDs and clothes among people they like and are often very organised, packing up boxes, filing papers away, perhaps writing letters of farewell.

They visit or phone their friends and often apologise to parents and siblings for things they may have said or done. At the same time there may be a marked improvement in their behaviour or mood.

At the other end of the spectrum, a young person who suddenly embraces booze and drugs with open arms and defiant daring, particularly if there has been no previous interest in this sort of excessive risk-taking behaviour, may well be on the verge of self destruction. Dangerous driving is often interpreted as supreme stupidity – it can also indicate that the young driver doesn't care if he lives or dies.

Other warning signs include:
- Not caring about how they look and poor hygiene
- Putting themselves down
- Being easily upset and constantly agitated
- Truancy from school or taking sickies from work
- Unusual habits such as not eating, or overeating and vomiting.

A previous attempt at suicide automatically puts a young person into a high risk category. A suicide attempt is any act or action that can lead to injury or death. The most obvious attempts are gunshots, overdosing on pills, carbon monoxide poisoning and razor or knife wounds. Less obvious attempts include self-harming behaviour such as carving initials into the body, burning themselves, drug and alcohol abuse and driving dangerously.

Tragically there are a few boys and girls who give no signs at all. They act on impulse, when they are suddenly overwhelmed. They just do it.

Unpremeditated suicide attempts are more common among young people from broken and unhappy homes and if their lives are saved in time, they need urgent and specific psychiatric treatment.

Young people who try to kill or hurt themselves desperately need help. The old-fashioned view that such behaviour is designed purely to draw attention, has become utterly unacceptable.

Of course they want attention – a suicide attempt is a cry of need, an acknowledgment that they can't cope with life. It's the responsibility of every one of us to help them. Their next attempt may be their last, in the worst of possible ways.

SPEAKING OF
JASON . . .

It's Saturday night at the Connors' crowded house and
STACEY, nineteen, is going out. Her boyfriend is on his way to
pick her up – he works at the mines with Peter and tonight's
a big night for their social club. Stacey has treated herself to a
scented bath to take the sting out of her burns ('Put in some
rose oil,' says her mother; 'Just a few drops,' calls Peter) and
now she lines up six bottles of perfume on the big table and
asks Lee to recommend the best scent for the night. Her face
is immaculately made up, her fair skin glows. She has pale
blonde hair, straight and shiny as cellophane, and round
spectacles. She laughs and squirts her mother with Red Door.
She has put on long black crepe trousers and a glittery top
and she wants to know if she looks okay. She does. Her
figure must be the envy of every girl in town.

Stacey's voice, when she sits down to talk, is solemn and
husky. It's going to be a great asset when she qualifies as a
librarian.

'When Jason was about thirteen, Mum and Dad put him on
a diet. I remember us walking together and he stopped off at
the shop and bought sausage rolls and Crunchie bars and we
were scoffing them on the way home. Suddenly we saw
Mum and Dad coming around the corner in the car. He
threw all the food away so they wouldn't see him eating. It
was so funny.

'He was a real boy, always off with his mates, riding bikes, bushwalking, that sort of stuff. He was pretty happy, but the boys at school used to call him Fatso. They were really cruel.

'I remember Jason going jogging when he was about fourteen. He would put on two garbage bags and lots of jumpers to try and sweat off the weight.

'The best times at our place are Christmases because we are all together, and birthdays. We always have dinner together and a cake. There are so many of us coming and going that often we miss each other, but at Christmas you know that nobody will be missing.

'When Jason was in his own house I used to go up and stay with him. We'd go shopping in the city; I'd help him choose the family's presents. He put money aside every week for presents but he never knew what our sisters wanted and whatever I said, he'd buy it. Sometimes we'd get videos and go home and watch them and talk and drink coffee.

'I never knew whether he smoked pot. He wouldn't have done it in front of me. He would have known I would have looked down on him for doing that.

'He had started getting very conscious of what he was eating. He never had junk food in the house any more. When we went out to eat I would order fish and chips and he would eat salad. I never diet myself. I just exercise – lots of aerobics and walking.

'I didn't think he was unhappy until one day when he came up to me, really upset, and he asked me if I thought he had lost heaps of weight. "Well, yes, you have," I said. I don't think he realised himself how thin he was getting. He was starting to look shorter and sort of shrunken. "Stacey," he said, "you are the only person who hasn't told me I look terrible." He was really angry. Normally Jason was such a placid person, always smiling. It was scary when he got upset and angry because it wasn't him.'

Peter tries to describe his eldest daughter before she arrives. 'A hippie type,' he says. 'Wears real tight shorts or long droopy dresses and riding boots without socks. Masses of bloody hair.' When she appears, graceful and erect despite the fact that her small daughter, Jessica straddles one narrow hip, Ceane's appearance is in remarkable contrast to her fair and red-headed siblings. Slightly built and slender, she has creamy coffee skin, a high, wide brow, enormous dark eyes and a torrent of black curls. What modesty prevented the proud father from saying, is that CEANE is strikingly beautiful.

She seems confident, articulate and animated, but her reminiscences are punctuated with bursts of nervous, uncertain laughter and her gaze wavers and drifts from time to time, when the remembering becomes painful.

'Charmaine and I used to hassle Jason all the time when we were kids. We'd hide under his bed and when he came in from the shower we'd jump out and laugh at him and he'd chase us out.

'As little kids we spent a lot of time up in the mountains, climbing the cliffs, exploring. If Mum knew what we did up there she would have killed us. We'd go up for whole days at a time, the three of us and a friend each and the dog. Jason was a bit more responsible than the rest of us. Mum and Dad had impressed on him that he was the eldest ...

'That's why he was allowed to ride his bike to school and I wasn't. Then he got a motorbike. He used to ride over to our nan's on it. They were very close – he practically lived there half the time. He was much closer to them than the rest of us were.

'When I was about thirteen he told us he had a different father to the rest of us. It was a hush hush business; it was never discussed. It made no difference to us. Deep down it would have worried him I think, but it would worry any normal person to a certain degree, wouldn't it?

'I know the kids at school used to call him a coon because that's what they called me, too. Any Aboriginal person goes through it at the start. When you get older it doesn't bother you any more because you stop worrying about what people say, you know? You accept what you are and you don't care what anyone else thinks of you. At least, that's what I did ...

'I mean so what if you are Aboriginal? It's supposed to be getting better for us now ... mind you,' – a great gurgle of breathless laughter – 'I don't know about *that* being true ...

'Jason was very accident prone. He was in a serious car accident about four years ago when he broke his sternum. Before that he broke his nose in the pool and he got hit by a truck when he was on his bike. He was always breaking his fingers.

'He wasn't the type to pick a fight but he would get into fights when it was a matter of protecting me or the others. I remember one time in particular when some boys stuck their finger up at me and I gave them the finger back and they ended up fighting Jason, even though it was really my fight, not his.

'It was part of his being such a perfectionist, I think. He was always very concerned when things went wrong and he stressed about it until he could do something to fix it.

'I left school in Year Eleven and I've worked in a few different jobs since then. I met up with this bloke who I've been with for seven and a half years. Two and a half years ago we had Jessica Rose. Now I'm doing a management training course at a drug and alcohol rehabilitation centre.

'I've been a marijuana smoker and when I first left school I dabbled in a bit of speed, but only for a short while. Jason used marijuana here and there. He didn't drink. We'd try and drag him into the pub but he'd say "nup", he didn't want to go. We'd say: "Okay but come and have a game of pool, ya don't have to drink."

'Jason was unique because although he wasn't weird or anything, he would never go up to a woman and hit on her like most men would. Men sort of hint and women respond if they want to. He wouldn't hint. I told him he was too nice. He had a lot of girls as friends but he never had a serious relationship. I think he started well with a couple of girls when he was younger but his mates took them off him ...

'He always wore a cap ...

'His house was absolutely spotless. He put all of us to shame.

'I know he had started travelling down to the city a lot and he was getting headaches. He told me he couldn't sleep at night and he was always tired. Something went wrong with his car and it cost him heaps of money to get it fixed. He was worried about work, too. He was sick of it. We would drop in on him and my boyfriend would try to talk him into leaving his job and getting into woodchopping or truckdriving with him.

'He was obviously going through a really bad time, which is why I feel really horrible in one respect. He had always called me Skinny Minny. This particular Saturday he came around to see me. I saw him walking down the street towards me and I thought: "Oh my goodness look how skinny Jason is. Here's the go. It's my chance to tease him back." So I called out: "Hi Skinny Minny!"

'The next day I found out he said to his friends: "I'm sick of this. When I was fat they called me Fatso. Now I'm thin they all call me Skinny." It was like he just couldn't please anybody and we were all driving him mad ...

'I actually attempted suicide once. I was pregnant, stressed out with worry ... I couldn't find any answers. I just didn't know what I wanted out of my life. I was pissed off about how I was always feeling down. I thought: "Stuff this. I'm going." I left a note for my boyfriend and got in my car and drove into the bush. I followed the dirt road, full of bumps and kangaroos and things, and I went up to the glow-worm tunnel. I didn't wear my seat belt, I just wanted to drag myself off the road and have an accident or something. That's how much I cared about myself at the time ...

'Trouble was, every time I got to a curve in the road, I couldn't do it. I kept turning the wheel at the last minute so I wouldn't crash.

'What got me out of it was I got into the tunnel and it was dark and I was scared being up there on my own. It was doomy, just like the thoughts I was having. I wasn't on drugs or anything at the time so the fear really got hold of me. I think if you are under the influence of drugs, you don't have enough sense to be frightened and that's what makes them so dangerous.

'While I was sitting there this big storm blew up, and it stormed all around my car, trees blowing and lightning striking and thunder and everything. It scared me so much. I turned my car around and started driving back down the road and then I saw this white kangaroo ... Well, I mean how many people see white kangaroos? To me it was like a sign from God. So I went home.

'I had sorted my own mind out by the time I got back. Trouble was, people were looking for me. The police were even looking for me. It was embarrassing. It was so embarrassing. Maybe some people go ahead and kill themselves because they have gone too far to go back and they can't bear the thought of what would happen if they changed their minds.

'I snapped out of it pretty fast and I never did anything like that again. When things had settled down, Jason said to me: "You silly girl. Don't you *ever* think of doing anything like that again. If you want to do that," he said, "you come and talk to me first".

'Later on I thought: "You hypocrite, Jason".'

It's Sunday morning and around the corner from the Connors' house, JOEL is looking after his baby son in a neatly renovated, rented cottage. He's a dark-haired, clean cut young man of twenty-six, a spray painter with a sweet smile. Joel is a nickname he earned in primary school; he was the tallest boy on the cricket team so they called him Joel Garner and the name, if not the game, stayed with him.

'Jason's sisters used to drive him mad. They used to bundle all their boyfriend problems onto him and he always felt he had to sort them out. It was good when he moved out of town and got his own place because he needed a bit of a break from his family.

'He didn't like it here in town. He hated the way everyone knew everyone else's business.

'Jason and I have been friends since infants school; he was always a bundle of laughs, always the one to give other kids something to smile about. He was a very funny man.

'He was a big boy. We played soccer together when we were thirteen and we had to practically push him around the field, he was that slow and heavy. Everyone took the mickey out of him but he got them back with his wit and humour.

'By the time we were all leaving school we had a big group, about twelve guys and we were pretty close, pretty tight. We went bushwalking, we went on rides in the mountains and later we drove up there. We were never bored. We did all that growing up stuff together – drank, smoked a bit of pot – even tried growing our own. Jason didn't drink after his twenty-first birthday, when we got him rotten. He said he didn't like what grog did to people.

'As a young man he was still the clown. He had a big heart. Whenever any of us had a problem we'd go and see him at his house.

'He would come around to my place and talk to me and my mum and my grandmother who has always lived with us. My dad died when I was real small and Mum was left with four little kids to look after. She says she stayed here because the people in the town were so good to her. Anyway, sometimes Jason would talk about finding his real dad. He really wanted to know who his real dad was but the idea of it frightened him.

'It was a bit of a shock when he found out he had an older brother, too. He had always thought the brother was his uncle.

'He used to love his job at Telecom but he hated it at the railways. He worked on phone lines and signals. The trouble was, he couldn't afford to leave it because he was paying off a loan on his car. He'd get mad with his mum if he needed to borrow money from her and she didn't have it. The thing was, he didn't get paid much unless he did heaps of overtime. He was really good at putting on a cheerful front but sometimes when I went up to see him he'd go off his head about work – once he had the dummy spat, that was it with Jason. He'd go right off.

'He was devoted to his nan and to his uncle, who had some sort of breakdown and couldn't look after himself. Jason would go and see them and give them a hand, get a fire going, shave his uncle, that sort of thing. But they both died.

'He was only really depressed in the last few weeks and I think a lot of it was down to losing massive amounts of weight. He did it properly, eating the right food and everything, but he hid what was happening to his body. Jason was always very good at hiding things. If you tried to talk about his weight with him he'd just get stroppy and go off.

'He was proud of being Aboriginal but he didn't talk much about it in case people thought he benefited from it. He joked about being confused about who he actually was. He said he was like a can of soup – fifty-seven varieties. I think it worried him deep down.

'Our mate Jack drew things real well and he did this cartoon of Jason with the Mabo flag tattooed across his chest. Jason laughed and laughed when he saw it.'

ABORIGINAL KIDS

Oh, we have benefited, we have been lifted
With new knowledge, a new world opened.
Suddenly caught up in a white man's ways
Gladly and gratefully we accept,
For this is necessity.
But remember, white man,
If life is for happiness,
You too, surely, have much to change.

From *Civilisation* by Oodgeroo of the tribe Noonuccal
(formerly known as Kath Walker)

Black boys can't cope.

Who can blame them? Given a choice of skin colour and heritage, how many of us would choose to be an Aboriginal Australian?

During the two hundred years since European settlement began in Australia, the native people who have been here for thousands of years have lost their freedom, their lands, and until very recently, many of their children. In their ignorance and without waiting to be asked, a precedent having already been set for them in North America and Africa, white men made themselves responsible for weaning Aborigines away from their culture, their religion and their way of life. Frequently with the best of intentions, often with religious zeal, sometimes through blind intolerance, cruelty and a deplorable absence of compassion or even common sense, Europeans have attempted to bring their version of civilisation to Aboriginal people.

As a result, for many years, Aborigines have been regarded as inferior to whites. They have been kept away from places where white people gather, and deprived of white people's rights and freedoms, yet they have been expected to learn to live like European Australians, adapting to the lifestyle, the religion, the customs, the food, the drink, the manners, and the values of the same people who have consistently shut them out.

There has now been a substantial change in the public attitude to black Australia. Shaming and shameful restrictions and injustices have been lifted. Aboriginals are being urged by the more successful and secure members of their race, and by sympathetic whites, to celebrate their origins, to show the world how proud they are to be Aboriginal Australians.

Some politicians would even have us all believe that it has become an advantage to be black in this country. Not too many white people would agree.

Even fewer Aboriginal people do.

More than any other group of young people in Australia, young Aboriginal men are experiencing enormous confusion about the role they are meant to play in a society to which they have never truly belonged. They are confused not only by what is expected of them as males but also by what is expected of them as males descended from a totally different culture to the one in which they find themselves.

Some have the need to radically affirm their Aboriginality because they feel excluded from the wider society. Others have the desire to radically disavow it. The middle can be a lonely place ... young people of mixed race are particularly vulnerable.

Among all young people throughout our society, self-harming talk, self-harming behaviour and dangerous risk-taking involving drugs and alcohol, have become a recognised way of articulating desperation, rage and helplessness. Nowhere is this so rife as it is in the Aboriginal community. For too many young Aboriginal men, the only solution to the problems of life is death.

The rate of suicide among Aboriginal and Torres Strait Islander men aged from fifteen to twenty-nine is believed to be more than double that of other young people. Figures are difficult to establish because of widespread under-reporting; even the Aboriginals themselves have little idea of how many of their boys are dying. However, government research suggests that for every thirty-four young white males (per 100,000 population) who take their own lives, at least seventy young black males are committing suicide. The number of deaths has seriously increased over the past decade.

The grim statistics do not relate to all Aboriginal people and certainly not to all age and gender groups. Some indigenous communities (though certainly not all), particularly those based on the traditional ways, have very few suicides. Aboriginal women have a slightly lower suicide rate than average.

The causes, issues and potential prevention programs relating to Aboriginal youth suicide are complex and controversial, as Professor Ernest Hunter, a specialist in cross-cultural psychiatry, explains.

'Imagine you are a young Aboriginal man. You come from a remote Aboriginal community. You left school at the statutory leaving age, having been absent for a third to a half of all school days, with a reading level of grade one or two. You then enter into a government program which pays you to do menial work two days a week for very little money without providing you with any of the skills you need to enable you to use the apparent free choice which our society is supposed to provide.

'You are going to feel angry and dispirited but you are probably not going to be able to put it into words. You are certainly not going to be able to use the political system to your advantage. You will be caught in a whole set of social circumstances that will continue to entrap you.

'This situation does not apply to all Aboriginal people, but it does apply to many.

'The resulting anger and indignation can be precipitated by very minor events – being refused money, the break up of a relationship, a minor insult. The next thing that happens is that you're dead.'

Professor Hunter compared the situation of a desperately unhappy young Aboriginal with that of a middle-aged white man. 'When an older European person is diagnosed as suffering from depression, he or she would be given medical help; their condition would be monitored for three weeks until the medication began working.

'When the situation involves an Aboriginal person, it's a matter of getting him through the twenty-four hours following the event which catapulted him into a state of distress. If he survives that time, he will probably be all right a week later.

'To address the underlying issues which brought about his distressed state requires intervention at a community level and is a much greater challenge.'

LOSING THEIR PLACE

When Australia was colonised by white Europeans, the Aboriginals lost more than their land. They also lost their place in society – the sacred and economic roles of Aboriginal men were seriously undermined.

'These had been extremely important roles,' said Professor Hunter. 'They were the way in which young men learned how to become socially privileged people in their community. The transition from one phase of life to another for males became very poorly defined.

'The same thing happened to the indigenous people in the US and Canada, through processes which were both planned (such as removal of children from their families, in order to turn them into something other than people of the culture from which they came) and unplanned (the experience of dislocation).

'Not only were young Aboriginals subjected to procedures which were supposed to be for their own good, they were then often mistreated, abused and sexually abused in the schools and settings to which they were sent.

'They were triply victimised in the sense that they were then made to feel responsible for what had happened to them. This had a serious effect on their personal integrity.'

Over the past thirty years, the white population has become very slowly more enlightened with regard to its indigenous people. The 1980s saw the Royal Commission into Black Deaths in Custody; most of the restrictions on Aboriginal people have now been lifted. Opportunities for the indigenous population are substantially greater than they have ever been, legislation is becoming less onerous and regulations less draconian. More Aboriginals are making their own unique mark on the achievements of the country.

Yet, at this crucial time, the rate of suicide among young Aboriginal men has leapt alarmingly.

'During the years that Aboriginal people lived under severe restrictions, there was a very clear structure surrounding them,' said Professor Hunter. 'They weren't accountable to themselves or to anyone else. The reasons for their circumstances were clear. People had done things to them. People had come and taken their children away. People had made them suffer, yet what they could do about it was limited.

'Then those limits were lifted and the wider society sat back and told them whatever their situation was, it was their own fault. They were given new freedoms, but the doors of opportunity frequently led into the cupboard of welfare dependence.

'Their "empowerment" is illusory. It has gone from a life of institutional dependency on mission stations with no rights, to institutional dependency on government subsidies with rights but few opportunities to build on them.'

During the sixties and seventies, massive and rapid changes occurred in Aboriginal communities; unemployment became rife but dole cheques put cash in people's hands. At the same time, unlimited amounts of alcohol were made available to them.

'Aboriginal people were not just attracted to alcohol,' said Professor Hunter. 'They were led to it by European people who saw a buck in selling grog to them.'

Another problem has been the absence of effective tribal and family influence. The role models which once existed for Aboriginal young people have been seriously compromised over the past thirty years, said Professor Hunter.

'The young Aboriginal men of the sixties and seventies were caught up in the chaos of change. Some ended up dying in accidents and violence, many spent their lifetime abusing alcohol. Relationships broke up. Their lives were profoundly affected; their capacity to provide an environment of stability for their children was compromised. The young people who are killing themselves in the eighties and nineties are the children of that generation.

'In a way, Aboriginal children are still being removed from their families. They are being removed into the criminal justice system. Their parents are still being removed from their role because of the consequences of substance abuse.'

'APPEALING' VIOLENCE

Because Aboriginal youths have not been given the tools to articulate their grievances, they have no means of seeking redress for the evil that has been done to them. They are, however, increasingly aware of the injustice their race has suffered.

Years ago, Aboriginals lived in ignorance of their situation. There was very little information about their plight getting out to the world, but there was even less information getting in. Life was fairly predictable and structured.

Now there is an awareness of what is going on; they realise their levels of disadvantage. Despite being told that they are now in charge of their own lives, the opportunities for most have not significantly improved. Yet they are expected to take responsibility.

'Many of them do,' said Professor Hunter. 'The dilemma is that at the same time there is the profoundly inhibiting effect of alcohol and drugs.'

Miserable, misplaced and angry with the world, young Aboriginals take out their desperation on themselves rather than on society. This is called 'appealing violence', a form of protest without obvious direction which results in them punishing themselves, initially through alcohol and drug abuse and, too often, through suicide.

Like any people who seek escape through excessive alcohol use, young indigenous people are prone to psychological difficulties which, when compounded by drug abuse (particularly marijuana) can result in psychosis.

DEATHS IN CUSTODY — PLANTING A DEADLY IDEA

'The Royal Commission into Aboriginal Deaths in Custody which began in 1987 did many good things,' said Professor

Hunter. 'However, the media coverage and public debate which surrounded the commission may have had unexpected consequences – including increasing the rate of suicide.

'When the interim report was released at the end of 1987, the Royal Commissioner, Justice Muirhead, pointed out that in comparison with non-Aboriginals, excessive numbers of Aboriginal people were *not* committing suicide in custody; the problem was that so many Aboriginals were in custody in the first place.

'Justice Muirhead then appropriately shifted the commission to an examination of underlying causes for the numbers of Aboriginals in gaol. Underlying causes don't sell newspapers or make interesting television, so interest in the issue faded.'

Unfortunately, much was made of the deaths in cells and lockups. Macabre jokes began circulating among the white population. Some white people genuinely believed that Aboriginals were killing themselves because they couldn't stand to be in confined spaces. (But Aboriginals have been being sent to gaol for nearly 200 years – the increase in suicides occurred only recently; around about the time, it should be noted, as drug use became prevalent.) The publicity which surrounded the subject of Aboriginal deaths in custody presented to desperate, disillusioned and susceptible people, a personal resolution to what in their moments of turmoil might have felt like irresolvable problems.

'From that time on we have had a really significant increase in suicides,' said Professor Hunter.

Compensation through education

While Aboriginal people have every right to the same range of clinical services as any Australian – or more access in terms of their needs – improved health services are unlikely to address the real issues behind the problem of Aboriginal youth suicide.

'This is not a third world country,' said Professor Hunter. 'Aboriginal people are not dying from starvation and other third world blights; they don't need barefoot doctors. They are dying from diabetes, heart disease, lung disease, alcohol, accidents and other lifestyle diseases. And suicide.

'The solution to the problem of Aboriginal youth suicide is certainly not more psychiatrists. There has to be a change in the circumstances of Aboriginal people, but that makes it a social justice issue, not just a health issue.

'Medical answers by and large are cheap – a new clinic here, a crisis centre there – the dollars mount up but in terms of comparing that with the investment that a social justice solution would require, it's significantly less. The difference is really doing what it takes to ensure educational outcome, employment equity, reconciliation and atonement.'

When it comes to the process of atonement, said Professor Hunter, there is still a long way to go.

'We've done reports on black deaths in custody, on stealing away the black babies, on racism – but there has to be more than that. It's been said that there are three elements to atonement. There is acknowledgment. There is restitution – giving back that which can be given back. Then there is compensation – for that which cannot be given back.'

Professor Hunter believes the most effective way to compensate indigenous Australians for all that they have lost would be to provide an education system which would genuinely advantage the next generation of Aboriginal young people.

'Education for Aboriginal people has been an unmitigated disaster. The plot has been lost in terms of output. Two-thirds of Aboriginals live in towns and cities, so it's not simply an issue of remoteness. Many kids are getting zippo. The exposure to the accoutrements of the good life reinforces the nature of their distress.

'Education is about providing the tools that enable real choices to be made. I'm not talking about assimilation. I'm talking about education as a means to providing control over one's life, including the very way being Aboriginal is understood.

'Let's not forget that in addition to the many Aboriginal people who are trapped in a cycle of distress, there are others who are similarly angry and indignant but who are lawyers and professionals; they don't kill themselves. They are frequently out there pushing for white bureaucrats to be responsible to international and national conventions and legislation. They can do that because they have the tools.'

WHERE IS THEIR HOPE?

Like young people everywhere, young Aboriginal people need hope. For Aboriginals, however, that hope is dependent on fundamental social change. The question is: can the government change the way people think?

Better still, can we change it ourselves?

How do you convince an unsympathetic public that when a young black man kills himself, he is not trying to attract attention to himself, nor is he making a political act of protest?

He is just giving up.

'I don't think any black kids are impulsively committing suicide as a conscious political act,' said Professor Hunter. 'They probably don't think about it in any systematic way, apart from the fact that on some level they are saying to the world: "Fuck you".'

Now brood no more
On the years behind you,
The hope assigned you
Shall the past replace,
When a juster justice
Grown wise and stronger
Points the bone no longer
At a darker race.

From *Song of Hope* by Oodgeroo
of the tribe Noonuccal (formerly Kath Walker)

Ernest Hunter is Professor of Public Health (Mental Health)
at the University of Queensland's Northern Clinical School in
Cairns. He has worked in Hawaii in the field of indigenous
mental health and in the Kimberley region of Western
Australia. Professor Hunter has carried out research into
Aboriginal and Islander populations in Cape York and the
Torres Strait Islands and has worked for the Redfern
Aboriginal Medical Service in Sydney.

MAZ: BEING VERY BAD

' I was the girl with the curl, you know? When I was good, I was very good but when I was bad I was BAD. I mean, seriously bad.

I started smoking at twelve and by Year Eight I was drinking and smoking dope – bongs mostly, made from the neighbour's hoses. We used to get the older kids to buy what grog we needed and we'd go down and get rotten at the oval or the Lookout Park. Lookout – that was a joke. You got a view of the arse end of all the unit blocks. This was mostly at night. I would just tell Mum I was going to one of my girlfriend's houses. At weekends I said I was sleeping over. She never let anyone sleep over at our place, no prizes for guessing why. So she was just as pleased to believe that I was getting invited out, I suppose.

I got rid of my virginity behind the toilets on the oval, when I was fourteen. I loved the feel of boys. They didn't smell like my father, all sickly sweet and clean. They smelled sweaty and hot and young and dirty. They cuddled you and kissed you and they'd make you feel really special for a while, but boys get sick of sex pretty quickly. Then they talk to you horribly and you wonder why you bothered. My girlfriends were more important to me at that stage. I had three best friends, and they all had problems. Two were from broken-up families and their mums had to work a lot and the other one was like me – her parents hated each other. Only it was worse for her because they hated her as well. I knew my parents didn't hate me. I just annoyed them because I wasn't, like, normal.

Sometimes we talked about killing ourselves. A few of the others had scars on their wrists where they said they had already tried. It was a bit of a cult thing, like who had tried the most and how many times. Mind you, some of them who just lived with their mums, I thought were quite lucky. At least they didn't have to listen to the rows or sit at the table feeling the tension in the atmosphere eat at your guts like acid. Sometimes I wondered why my father didn't just go. My mum wouldn't, of course. That wouldn't be Doing the Right Thing. But the old man – if he wanted to drink himself silly and bonk half the city, why didn't he just leave us and go and live somewhere else?

I hated the double standard at home. We *weren't* a nice family. We *weren't* happy. It was such hypocrisy. It was all such a big lie.

Trouble is, in a way, I was just as bad. You're probably wondering how I got away with all this mucking up and the truth is, I was a brilliant liar. But I also did a lot of Right Things at school and that pleased them – my parents I mean. I kept getting good marks, I was elected house captain – that was easy, so many kids owed me. I was even elected to the Student Representative Council and I went on this trip up to Sydney and we stayed in a student hostel. I met this guy who was also a great pretender, like me, and we sneaked out and we found some *very* good dope, not to mention a few sweet secrets of our own, if you know what I mean.

By the time we were sixteen we could easily sneak into the pubs and we could get better drinks. Everyone had casual jobs, either at Maccas or as checkout chicks, so money wasn't really a problem. I worked in a doughnut shop. Some of my friends were getting into the drugs in a big way by then – it's easier when you work. I hated cigarettes so I just stuck to the dope and the drinks myself. And the boys. I was dying to fall in love with somebody. I knew that would make me happy. Anyway, finally I met Jake. He worked with me at the doughnut shop, but he was a bit younger and at first I didn't take a lot of notice of him. But it turned out he really really loved me and he was so sexy because he was young and keen, you know, and caring. I didn't even have to be drunk to enjoy doing it with Jake. We started talking about running away together and we made all our plans. We saved up even. It wasn't just some hare-brained scheme or anything.

The night we were meant to go I arrived at the train station first. I waited and waited. After three hours sitting on the platform I figured Jake had chickened out on me. Smart, hey? You can see I'm not just a pretty face! You can't imagine how I cried. I cried and cried and cried. It's a wonder that platform didn't just float away. A few people gave me odd looks but nobody said anything. Girls cry a lot on railway stations in the city.

I went anyway. I caught a train as far as it went and then I started hitching. Two truck drivers, one nice, the other not so, took me all the way up to Sydney. The yuck driver wanted to feel me up but I just got out of there and ran. I caught another train into the city and I went to sleep in a bus shelter. Some cops woke me up and I said I had fallen asleep by accident and was on my way to my auntie's. They left me alone, but then this other guy came and hung around. It was real early in the morning of my second day away from home. He looked a bit shifty but all he wanted was a light and then he asked me if I was looking for a refuge. I thought that was a pretty good idea at the time so he told me where to go.

I had heard how you can get this money from the government, this allowance, if you want to live away from home. The people at the refuge told me all about it but to qualify I had to get my parents to sign this thing saying they were not willing to be responsible for me any more, because they couldn't control me, or something like that.

Well, I rang them up. Pretty stupid, hey? Of course there wasn't a hope in hell of them signing. I suppose I knew that, really, but I still called. I kept thinking about Edward and Jilly, and how worried they would be.

It turned out that Jake had oh-so-sweetly spilled his cowardly little guts to *his* mother and she'd been going off about it all. Mum couldn't believe what this woman was telling her! The woman said I was a tramp, the school hole. I can just imagine Mum saying in her best voice that no child of hers would behave like *that*.

They *all* came up to get me. Can you believe it? They came in the car. They packed me up and put me in and nobody spoke to me all the way home. Twelve hours on the road and nobody spoke. I thought of requesting a nice version of *A Hard Day's Night*, with harmony, but I wasn't game.

When we got home Jilly told me she had been frightened and that she had missed me. My parents never mentioned it again. They behaved as if it just hadn't happened.

Oh, except they made me give up my job. I suppose they worked out that's how I could afford to run away. And about a week later Edward suggested that I could see the school counsellor. Mum just gave him a pained look and walked out of the room.

As if we would tell anybody we weren't perfect.

Two months later we moved to Sydney. I was just going into my final year of high school and I had to take different subjects if I was going to do the Higher School Certificate, so it wasn't an easy change for me. Edward stayed in Melbourne. He was at university by then and it would have mucked him up. Nobody worried about how much I was being mucked up.

You'd have thought with a fresh start in a nice big city, everything would have improved. In fact, things got worse between my parents. Our father didn't travel any more and their rows were right there, in our faces, every night and all weekend. He was getting a red puffy look about him, with all the grog. He wasn't as pretty as he used to be. Whenever he had a go at me about all my ear rings and the naval ring and the body piercing generally, I told him he was no painting either. That made him madder than anything. You wouldn't believe what he called me when Mum wasn't listening.

The new school was okay. I made friends pretty quickly, as usual. I let Sooz be my best friend because she had really bad skin and she walked sort of funny and you could tell she had never had a best friend in her life. I told her the whole story of my life, and all my problems, and she told me hers. I knew she would be a safe person to take home, too. When I took pretty girls home our father used to try to flirt with them; he always had to stroke them or touch them. It made me want to vomit.

I also got a new boyfriend, Danny. Then I met Danny's best mate, who was a year older than us and had left school. He came on to me pretty strong. Gazza was his name, we were Gazza and Maz which sounded pretty cool. He was gorgeous, tall and blonde. My new friends said he had been through everyone in the school and he wasn't a one-girl guy. I didn't know what I had done to get on to such a cool boy but I made the most of it. After a while I was getting those same looks from the other girls at school that I used to get in Melbourne – they were so jealous and they spread stuff about me, but I didn't care. I felt a bit bad about Danny though, and I tried to get him and Sooz together.

You'd have thought I would have just about run out of bad things to do by now but I still hadn't got pregnant. When I found out this had finally happened to me, I wasn't all that shocked. I had never taken any precautions and I suppose it was in the back of my mind that it would be nice to have a baby to love. I mean it really would. I have always loved babies and little kids. They are so uncomplicated and soft and cuddly.

I don't know how Mum knew. She was away all day every day and the only conversation we ever had started with her saying: 'Have you done your homework?' but somehow she guessed. She came into the bedroom one night and asked me if I was pregnant. I said probably, but it didn't matter because I was in love. She turned around and went out.

Then my father came in and told me we were going for a little drive. We drove to the lookout and parked and he said: 'Your mother is going to kill herself. She will probably kill Jilly as well, to save her any more misery. I hope you are happy now.'

I've been living with those words of his for a long time.

That night I cut my wrists really deeply but the door lock in the bathroom didn't work and Jilly came in. She screamed at the sight of all the blood and ran and told Mum of course. Mum just came in with her face whiter than mine, and bandaged up my wrists and drove me to the medical centre. She said to me: 'You can't do anything without making more trouble for all of us, can you?' I was sobbing my heart out, you know, tears and snot everywhere, and I blubbered: 'It would be better for me to die than you,' but she just looked even angrier. 'I don't know what you're talking about,' she said. 'I have no intention of dying and neither do you.'

I had a feeling it would be a long time before this one bad thing became a funny family story.

The people at the medical centre knew what was going on of course, and they told Mum I needed to see a counsellor and she promised to take me. I asked her about it when we got home and she said: 'Let's deal with one thing at a time.'

She was talking about the baby.

After that I just went on automatic pilot. I did everything I was told. They took me to see a doctor I didn't know and two weeks later we drove to a clinic somewhere close to the city. I did ask if I could take my doll, Bimbo Elizabeth with me for company. My mother told me not to be so melodramatic.

They dropped me off and I went in alone and waited in the waiting room and read *Dolly* magazine. It was an article about contraception.

Then they called me in and gave me a local anaesthetic and took away my baby. They told me lie down for an hour, which I did. Then I got up and got dressed and went down in the lift. My father was waiting in the lobby. I joined him and we got in the car with my mother. For once it was just the three of us. Their biggest concern this time was that Jilly should never find out. Jilly had been upset enough by the wrist slashing incident. She had to be protected from further trauma. Never mind about my trauma! We had another long silent journey home. That night we went to our cousins' place for tea – Mum had one brother in Melbourne and one in Sydney and they both had kids. I liked the Melbourne cousins but the Sydney brother had three girls and they were nerds. I mean, they were nice enough, but they went to church and youth group and that – not my scene at all. You could tell they liked Jilly heaps more than me, even though I could always make them laugh themselves sick. Anyway, the grownups just pretended everything was normal. I couldn't eat my dinner, which was unusual.

This incident was also too serious to become a funny little anecdote; it was never spoken of again. I went back to school the next week but it was a bit different. The principal was very nice to me. I was called into his office and he and the school counsellor, Mrs James – that's Diana – told me what a great student I was and how I had tremendous potential. The principal was a real slime but I liked Mrs James. She had a bit of a twinkle in her eye, you know, like the mother in 'Home Improvements'? They said if I had any problems I could talk to her, if I wanted to. From all this I gather someone had told them about the abortion. It must have been my father, although that seemed weird. No way could it have been my mother.

Anyway, they were so nice, and so was Sooz of course and funnily enough, so was Danny. Gazza disappeared, absolutely disa-bloody-peared. Bag and baggage. He had lived with his parents in a rented flat but it was vacant when I finally plucked up my courage and went to find him. I think my Dad might have had something to do with it. He knew some pretty weird people.

Mrs James used to give me a wave and a grin when she saw me, so one day I went to see her and we had a bit of a chat. That's when she suggested I start writing about my feelings.

To please Diana I put my head down for a while and I did really well in the HSC; not as well as Edward of course, but better than you'd expect. I could have gone to university but I didn't want to – my father's head was swollen enough, why give him another reason to brag about something that was nothing to do with him?

I never felt really happy again after they took my baby, you know? There was no point in talking to Diana about it because I knew *exactly* why I was miserable. I never mentioned it and she never asked.

Mum got me this job in a dress shop. She knew the manager. Some of my teachers were horrified but I just said I was taking a year to consider my options. Funnily enough, Mum didn't force the issue at all. She obviously didn't think I was good enough for uni. Meanwhile, things on the home front were really horrible. Dad had never hit Mum before, I don't think, but now he did. He smacked her face, at least twice. Protecting Jilly from trauma seemed to have fallen by the roadside. It came to a head because he had started another affair with someone at his office and he talked about it quite openly, comparing her favourably with Mum.

Sometimes when he drove me to work he picked this woman up on the way and it made my skin crawl having to pretend I didn't know what was going on. He would list off to her all his kids' greatest achievements. He always had to be selling something, even if it was *us*.

I was worried about it and I was always scared that Mum would kill herself, like he said that time, and maybe Jilly, too. Thinking about it, Mum would never have done that. Say what you like, she never gave in.

The best thing in my life was Danny. He didn't go to university either; he went to work for his Dad in his video shop and he was doing really well. Even though we had a rocky start, with the Gazza thing, he really loved me. He also knew all about me, so I didn't have to hide anything. Not that I was ever one for hiding anything, but you know what I mean. We could be totally honest with each other.

Danny was the nicest boyfriend I ever had and we didn't even have a sexual relationship. My mother, of all people, told me I should go to the doctor and get a prescription for the pill. I just kept staring at the television as if she wasn't there. But I really wasn't interested after having that abortion and Danny didn't seem to mind just having a kiss and lots of cuddles. We saw each other after work but Danny had to work every weekend.

I hated weekends. You can't imagine how horrible it was at home with just the four of us. Edward hardly ever came home. It might surprise you if I said my mother had a great sense of humour and in the past, when Dad was away on his travels, she used to tell a few family jokes and funny stories. Now there was never any laughter. The tension was hideous. Then one of them would do or say something and everything would explode into open warfare. Jilly spent all her time in her room.

If I wasn't seeing Danny or at work, I just watched television or I stayed in bed and tried to sleep. I was always tired. Mum noticed and she got some sleeping tablets from the doctor. She said they were for her and she kept them in her room but she gave one to me when I needed one. Honestly, Mum must have thought I was so stupid. As if I didn't know why she kept them locked away. The joke was, I found the prescription one day when I was looking for change in her handbag. There were repeats on it. I kept it. Just to show her she couldn't control me. Maybe to give her a fright. Anyway I kept it.

I hated the way I looked. I had my hair cut really short on top and shaved at the sides like a boy's; it really shocked my father and he stopped giving me a lift to work because he didn't want his girlfriend to know he had such a weird daughter. It didn't fit in with his story that his children were brilliant and attractive but his wife was a shrew. I also started getting really fat. People say: 'You're not fat, just cuddly,' but I started eating heaps. Sooz was the same. She was having huge problems with her mother as well. A few times we pigged out and then tried making ourselves sick, but it didn't work for me. I love food and it loves me. It just didn't want to come out. Sooz was better at it than me.

I was just so tired all the time and I used to think a lot about the baby, the one they took away. Danny was so sweet, he was always trying to cheer me up. He said when we were married, we could make another baby. Then Danny had this incredibly cool fabulous *wicked* idea! He said we should get engaged and get a house and move in together! Wow! I was so excited. I couldn't believe Danny wanted to spend the rest of his life with me, but he did. He had saved up a lot of money already and I was saving too. We decided to put a deposit on a block of land. We applied for a loan. It was the first step to building our own house and getting married and having a baby. Maybe lots of babies.

I was going to get out. I was going to get away from it all. It was the only thing that kept me going, really, the thought of moving away from the Unit of Destruction – that's what I called our Sydney flat in my head – the thought of escaping and finding some – you know – happiness and stuff. We were really sweating on that loan coming through. I kept thinking: 'Please let it happen and then I'll be good. I'll be *very* good. I'll Do the Right Thing, everyone will be pleased with me.'

'SHOULDN'T SOMEONE BE HELPING THEM?'

What sort of someone? Who are the experts in the treatment of suicide? Where do you find them? Even if you know of a good counsellor, how do you get a young person to agree to a consultation?

Imagine suggesting to your child, your brother, your sister, your friend, that it might be an idea for them to make an appointment with a suicide prevention specialist. It's not like seeing a dermatologist for a rash, or getting a referral from an ear, nose and throat doctor for an allergy test.

And yet, seeing a doctor is often an obvious and simple first step to helping a young person who is showing signs of serious depression.

GOING TO THE DOCTOR

When they were little, and they got sick, Mum took them to the doctor. Now they've grown up and they feel so bad they want to die, but maybe they are just sick. So they take themselves to the doctor, because doctors can make things better. Can't they?

According to clinical psychologist, Jon Pfaff, up to eighty percent of young people who engage in suicidal behaviour have been to see their doctor in the previous month. Other estimates put the figure at forty percent.

Whatever the numbers may be, the sad news is that many doctors miss the signs.

This is not surprising when rarely do troubled young people tell their local general practitioner that they feel depressed; they are even less likely to admit to being suicidal. They are more likely to come about acne or mysterious pain, weight gain, loss of appetite or sleep problems – almost anything other than the real reason they need help.

Jon Pfaff is project manager for the National General Practice Youth Suicide Prevention Project which is based in Western Australia. As a result of the escalating rate of mental illness (usually depression and anxiety) in the community, he recommends that all young people coming into general practitioners' surgeries be screened for psychological problems. 'When any level of distress is discussed and acknowledged by a young person, it should alert the GP to the possibility of suicide,' said Jon Pfaff, 'and he should raise the issue.

'The GP should ask for permission when changing the discussion from physical concerns to psychosocial issues and before asking sensitive questions about sex, substance use and suicidal thoughts,' said Jon Pfaff. Because a negative reaction by the doctor to any information given can increase the patient's distress, it's essential to establish a mutually respectful relationship before any help is given.

In their manual, *Managing Youth Suicidal Behaviour: A guide for general practitioners and community health personnel* (Commonwealth Department of Human Services and Health, 1996) authors Stephen J. Edwards and Jon Pfaff recommend a four step scheme aimed at prevention and intervention for potentially suicidal patients. They call these steps the 'four Rs'.

The four step rule for doctors

1. Recognise the signs – identify the warning signs that can lead to youth suicide
2. Raise the issue – encourage disclosure of suicidal ideas

3. Risk assessment – determine the youth's current level of risk and the urgency of clinical intervention
4. Respond – management and prevention

Jon Pfaff said doctors should never be afraid to discuss suicide openly with young people. 'The benefits of the information gained far outweigh any potential risk of precipitating a suicide,' he said. 'By coming to a GP a young person is indicating a need for help. In fact, this may be the only occasion they will have to talk about their situation.'

He warned GPs never to swear secrecy about suicidal plans; instead, limits of confidentiality could be discussed with the patient.

General practitioners need to develop a much greater awareness of the problem of youth suicide; they should also be familiar with all local services which can be made available to young people in crisis and to their families.

Unfortunately all of this takes time, a commodity which in many doctor's surgeries, is in very short supply. In many cases, doctors send young people off to different agencies which in turn refer them on to others. One of the biggest problems facing GPs is the time it takes to see a case through from the first tentative visit to the stage where genuine long term help is being provided.

IS THERE ANYTHING *WE* CAN DO?

Despite the sensitivity of the issue, Margaret Appleby, from the Rose Foundation, said family and friends can play a vital part in preventing death by suicide. She believes many suicides are preventable and what is needed is a greater degree of care and understanding both in the family and in the community. 'For too long it's been taboo to talk about suicide,' she said. 'It's time to break the silence. We all have what it takes to do something to prevent these tragedies.'

Many young people with strong connections to their families will still talk to their parents when they are deeply troubled. However, some parents may not be aware how much their comments and attitudes have hurt their children, or how badly they have been misunderstood. Parents can also be handicapped by the fact that changes in their children are less obvious when they see them every day; it's not always easy to discern the difference between teenage angst and suicidal behaviour.

Some parents put up barriers which prevent young people from confiding their distress. The terrible stigma which is attached to suicide means many adults blank the possibility out of their minds. In the words of bereaved mother Ruth Anderson, the thought that it could happen in their family frightens them to death. As for counselling – everyone might think there was something wrong.

The trouble is, everyone might be right.

Many young people are more likely to tell their troubles to a friend. It is also possible they will speak to a friend's mother or father, a respected teacher, a coach, a youth group leader or perhaps their minister or priest.

Whether you are a parent, a relative, an older person or a close friend, by listening you can destroy a disturbed young person's first reason for ending it all – the claim that nobody cares.

'There are three golden rules for anybody who has to deal with a suicidal person and particularly, a suicidal young person,' said Margaret Appleby.

'First, be a friend. Let them know you care.

'Second, don't be afraid to talk to them about their pain and distress and to listen to them. People on the brink of suicide need somebody to talk to, somebody who won't judge them or make them feel guilty or ignore them or trivialise their problems. All you have to do is listen.

'Third, after establishing a connection with a suicidal young person, talk to them about seeing a health care professional and if possible, *go with them* to see that person, while continuing to support them at a personal level.

'Never decide you can continue to counsel a suicidal young person entirely on your own. Even professionals working in the field have to be part of a team. But it may be a long time between consultations and support from home is as important as support in the consulting rooms or surgery. Success usually depends on the combined efforts of family, friends and health workers and it may take a long time.'

KITCHEN COUNSELLING

When ordinary people provide personal support for desperate people, it's sometimes called 'kitchen counselling'. For some people, communication comes more naturally than for others, but when suicide is threatened, there are a few rough rules to follow.

Margaret Appleby advised against offering advice, relating your own experiences in similar situations or thinking up solutions. 'Just listen. Establish a rapport with them by listening. Eventually, with your support and sympathy, you want them to find their own solutions.'

Lecturing suicidal people about their responsibilities is usually a waste of time. Telling them how much their loved ones will suffer if they take their life, reminding them of people they love (their sister's new baby, their invalid mother) or events they wouldn't want to miss, is not usually helpful when they are truly desperate.

'It's that tunnel vision again,' said Margaret Appleby. 'All they can focus on is their own emotional pain. They can't comprehend how anyone else may feel. They can't see sideways. They can only see themselves.'

Beware of minimising their problems. When his girlfriend dumped him, one boy's mother told him there were plenty more fish in the sea. He killed himself. The mother of a boy who told her he was thinking of committing suicide remarked this would save her a lot of money on muffins. Now bereaved, she would give anything never to have said those words. *(Yet what parent would blame her?)* It's hard enough for some young people to talk about their problems; it's near impossible if they feel that the person in whom they are confiding doesn't understand.

Nothing can replace the interest and sincerity of a loving parent, a sibling or a good friend. Once the lines of communication have been opened, and the troubles recognised and identified, the light at the end of the tunnel of despair may grow brighter with each passing day.

The last thing anyone should do after listening to a desperately unhappy young man or woman is to suggest that the two of you go straight to the hospital to get help. This is only necessary if the young person is likely to die – if they have already harmed themselves.

If you believe professional support *is* required, talk about it. You will probably have to explain that the two of you can't solve such serious problems on your own. Offer to help find an experienced professional who will believe in your young person, who can be trusted to listen and care.

Unfortunately, counselling is still widely misunderstood in Australian communities. People who 'give it a go' and feel no better after one session declare that it doesn't work. It may not be for everyone, but it's important to realise that counselling is not like taking a pill to get rid of a headache in half an hour. It is meant to be continuous and, for deeply troubled people, it may take months or even years before they have talked their way out of intense anxiety and into self-knowledge and peace of mind.

The advantage of talking to a counsellor rather than a friend (ideally, it's good to have both) is that you can keep saying the same things to a counsellor, without worrying about boring them witless and without having to listen to their problems in return.

Counselling is often prevented from working because of family influence. The stigma of mental illness is such that the parents may say: 'You're better now, you don't need that any more'. On the other hand, some parents who plead for professional help don't get it. Their own despair and helplessness is shunted aside. They may even be told it is them, not their child, who is neurotic.

Kids are good at covering up.

Where the rot really sets in is in the search for the right kind of counsellor. How do you find such a person? Where do you go? How much will it cost? By the time you have found someone, will the troubled teenager still be willing to submit to professional help?

In theory, assistance should be available from any local general practitioner, the adolescent unit at your nearest public hospital or your local community health centre. Look in the local community listings of the telephone directory. Suicide crisis lines are available in most areas. If the young person is still at school, the student counsellor may be able to refer you to a suitable source. A useful resource for young people who have left school are the social workers at the Department of Social Services. Counselling is also available from Relationships Australia (some areas offer RAPS, a specialist service for youth) and from the major churches, including the Salvation Army, Centacare, the Uniting Church (Unifam in NSW) and the Anglican Church (Lifeworks in Victoria). Organisations employing large numbers of people sometimes offer counselling services to employees' family members as part of their employee assistance programs. A list of counselling agencies, both public and private, can also be found in the Yellow Pages of the telephone directory. (Look up 'counselling: marriage, family and personal'.)

In practice, the availability of counsellors varies enormously, as do their work loads, their attitudes and the fees they charge. Some services, especially those at public hospitals, are free to young people. Government funded services may charge scaled rates or be means tested. Private counselling can cost up to $100 per visit.

'If a young person feels that the doctor, psychologist, counsellor – whoever it is – does not understand them or their problem, they should tell them so, and go,' said Margaret Appleby. 'They must find someone they can trust and who believes in them. That's another reason why it's a good idea for you to go with them, at least on the first visit.'

If at first you don't succeed ... ring around. Talk to people. Like good hairdressers and plumbers who turn up when they say they will, effective counsellors are often found by word of mouth.

It's not only prejudice and a bias against young people's moods which is limiting the support available to depressed adolescents. A shortage of funds, staff and time may render some services futile, to say the least. Currently, the health system, for many reasons, is letting down a lot of people.

You might have to keep up the kitchen counselling for quite a while.

Margaret Appleby has been working in the field of suicide prevention for many years. A Lifeline Director with a background in special education, and a specialist in crisis intervention counselling, in 1989 she established Rose Education, a publishing company which provides books and resources on loss, grief and suicide prevention.

The Rose Foundation was cofounded by Margaret Appleby, Gail Kilby and a group of people concerned with giving suicide prevention a higher profile in the community. The organisation dedicated to the prevention of suicide through the education of a wide variety of community groups, ranging from clergymen and doctors to teachers, health professionals, parents and students in schools. Support for those bereaved by suicide, through literature and group and individual counselling, is also a vital part of the foundation's work. With the assistance of trained counsellors and educators, Rose now operates in Queensland, Victoria, Tasmania, South Australia and New Zealand as well as New South Wales.

WHAT *WE* CAN DO WHEN SOMEONE THREATENS TO SUICIDE?

Hearing the Cry, by Margaret Appleby and Margaret Condonis, and published by Rose Education, is probably the best guide on suicide prevention available in Australia today. This extract explains what parents or indeed any of us can do if we believe a young person we know and probably love is contemplating suicide:

* Talk about it openly. Ask them if they feel so bad that they are thinking of hurting themselves.
* Listen to them. Watch their non-verbal behaviour.
* Tell them that if they need help, you are there for them.
* Offer to go with them to get help.
* Tell them you don't want them to get hurt or die because you will miss them.
* Take time to listen and be with them – time is a precious gift to give.
* Consult a professional if you are concerned about a young person's behaviour.

GARY: A LETTER FROM HIS DAD

To Whom it May Concern.
Gunnedah, NSW

I would like to comment on the delivery of mental health care in New South Wales.

I make these comments in the wake of the death of my son, Gary, who took his life in Mosman Bay in April, 1994, at the age of twenty-two, after an extended period of deep depression. For his family, having to cope with the onset and gradual deepening of his disorder was a new and bewildering experience and exposed what we regard as flaws in the mental health system and the delivery of care.

The Report of the National Inquiry into the Human Rights of People with Mental Illness says in its conclusion: 'It is clear … that the cost of mental illness in terms of human lives and suffering is enormous. In addition to the pain suffered by consumers, these costs include disruptions to family lives and sometimes unbearable pressures on other family members who feel powerless to assist the person who is ill'.

I would like to refer particularly to depressive mood disorders which are more widespread but less visible than schizophrenia. Depressive mood disorders are deep and often smouldering conditions, not obvious to the general community, nor even to health professionals, but a disturbing fact of life to family and close friends. The problem is compounded by the fact that the sufferers are often able to muster a bright and optimistic face for the medical profession, in order to escape treatment.

In the case of my son Gary, there was evidence of some psychological disturbance in adolescence which I believe was partly attributable to his sexual molestation at the age of fourteen by an adult male. His mental state was characterised by the excessive use of drugs, an episode of anorexia followed by a bout of bulimia, a period of obsession with study, followed by extreme listlessness and difficulty in motivating himself to study and doubts about his sexuality. His condition was frequently reflected in severe mood swings, from an euphoric state to one of deep gloom and despair, a state which began to accelerate in the last few years of his life.

Gary made two unsuccessful attempts on his life. In October, 1992, he overdosed on paracetamol while intoxicated and was admitted to a Sydney hospital.

This was the first time that any member of my family had been involved in any way with mental illness or the care of the mentally disturbed. It was new territory for us and quite disturbing to think that Gary had tried to end his life, even though we had been aware for some time of his depressed state of mind. He appeared to respond well to treatment but within a few months there were recurring episodes of depression and instances of psychological disorder, culminating in his very emotional revelation of his homosexuality in 1993.

My wife and I were amazed to hear so often from the health professionals that Gary was 'not mentally ill'. We were told that his depression and despondency did not constitute mental illness. It was very hard for us to reconcile this with Gary's preoccupation with death, his constant referral to suicide and his obsessive views on the state of society. He cared too deeply and thought too much, railed against injustice and saw greed and selfishness everywhere he looked. He talked more and more of finding his soul and going to a better and more beautiful place. It was our feeling that if all of this did not constitute mental illness, we did not know what did.

Very early in 1994 Gary's behaviour became even more irrational and the doctor who had treated him at the hospital arranged for a regional mental health counsellor to see him. The counsellor arranged for his scheduling to a mental health unit in Tamworth, but although Gary was there briefly, he refused all treatment. The family doctor and two Tamworth psychiatrists confirmed that he was very much at risk of suicide.

On the second occasion on which he tried to take his life, Gary was again living in Sydney. There was the familiar build up to an emotional breakdown – phone calls home with despair in his voice, his disillusionment with everything. I spoke to him late on the night of February 6 and I had the feeling that he was on the verge of a suicide attempt. Early the next morning I received a phone call, advising that he had tried to gas himself in a friend's car.

He was admitted to hospital – not the same one as before – initially as a medical patient.

The next day my wife travelled to Sydney and spoke to a female specialist who told her she had 'good' news. Gary was not mentally ill – he simply had personality disorder and was only trying to draw attention to himself. This information was repeated to us both over the next few days. We found it inconceivable that a person who had just made a serious attempt on his life could not be regarded as 'mentally ill'.

Four days later Gary, my wife and I met a senior staff specialist. As Gary had consistently refused any form of treatment, it was the impression of my wife and I that because he was not cooperative, the system felt there was nothing that could be done for him. It is hard for me to describe how desperate we felt about this. I remember saying to the doctor: 'Do you mean to say that only a few days after a near successful attempt on his life, Gary walks out of here into the community and we have to take our chances with him?' The doctor replied: 'That's right'.

The family was left to fend for itself, without any background experience in coping with Gary's condition. With hindsight, we should have more aggressively sought treatment for our son, at the hospital and when he came home. But not unnaturally we had become disillusioned with the system and lacked confidence in it. In country areas too, there are very few community-based support services for the mentally ill. Our town, Gunnedah, doesn't even have a resident mental health counsellor, although it has a population of 10,000 people.

Another problem is the ability of many mentally ill people to present well at psychiatric assessment interviews or to general practitioners. This was certainly the situation with Gary. There were no suicidal declarations or signs of psychosis at any time he was assessed. Our opinion was not considered.

I believe there should be more emphasis on the pattern of events leading up to the crisis. If a person makes an attempt on his life, doesn't that indicate a serious problem, no matter how well the person presents at the interview afterwards? There was no effort made to change Gary's attitude to treatment. We received no counselling on ways to deal with crises which might arise. We became the primary care-givers with no training, other than recent experience, to guide us.

Surely, even if a mentally ill person is denying that he needs help, someone should have the responsibility of ensuring that he gets the treatment he needs to get well. The health professionals seem to think that their hands are tied by the Mental Health Act. If that is the case, what use is that Act? Shouldn't it be amended?

I do not believe our situation is in any way unique. I have learned that it is a common cry. There should be a higher level of expertise in the psychiatric field to recognise and treat conditions like Gary's. Hundreds of thousands of people are suffering major depressive illness and there are, apparently, no specialist services or facilities for them.

I know that mental health care has moved away from the asylum era, when people were thrown into custody, segregated and isolated. That, of course, is entirely acceptable. But in the light of my experience, it seems that the Mental Health Act now enshrines the liberty of the sufferer above all else, at the expense of the people who know better than anyone else that their family member desperately needs help. Families are in the front line of the battle over mental illness and they feel frustrated and helpless when the person they love has lost touch with reality to the extent that he or she does not have sufficient insight to know that treatment is needed. It seems that the decision is entirely taken out of the hands of the family and left to the sufferer and 'the system' which is only too willing to allow that process to continue.

Their message to us is that you can't help those who won't help themselves. But if they are too ill to help themselves, what is to become of them?

I have felt an overpowering urge to put my thoughts on paper, because Gary was an exceptional person. He was too sensitive, too caring, experimented too much in life and eventually lost his way. But through all his troubles, he was someone of whom I was very proud and his loss is hard to bear.

I write in the faint hope that someone in authority will see that parents have rights too.

Ron McLean

June, 1994

Gary McLean committed suicide two months after being discharged from hospital into the care of his mother, Judy, and his father, Ron, the editor of the local newspaper. The second of four children, Gary was a mischievous and lovable child and a junior tennis champion. As a teenager he was popular, gregarious, strong and healthy (until the effects of his illness took their toll). He earned a tertiary entrance ranking of ninety-three in the Higher School Certificate and was studying psychology at university at the time of his death. In a letter to his parents before his second suicide attempt he wrote: 'There is too much pain in others for me to be happy'.

THE SYSTEM

Every family interviewed for this book – and there were many whose individual stories do not appear here – felt let down by the government health system. Faced with the horror of their children's suicide attempts and the realisation that their sons or daughters were deeply depressed, their pain and confusion was intensified by the fact that the professional help and support they needed was either difficult to find, unsympathetic, inaccurate in its diagnosis, rushed, clumsy, frightening, disjointed or expensive. Or all of the above.

'It's amazing how resourceful and exhausted some parents become,' said youth suicide prevention specialist, Barry Taylor. 'You work your way down the list of suggested support organisations and in a lot of cases, they've tried them all.'

The professional people most likely to be dealing with troubled adolescents are general practitioners, counsellors at community health centres and (depending on the degree of mental illness) psychiatrists, psychologists and social workers at public hospitals.

There are also psychologists at private clinics; for some families, the fees are beyond their means.

Parents who brought their (usually adolescent or adult) children to hospital following a critical event such as an attempted suicide, complained not only about a lack of caring staff but about being neglected themselves. While the young person may have been treated, counselled, quickly sedated and briskly saved in a room somewhere down the corridor, the parents spent agonising time alone. When their adolescent was returned to them they had no idea how to treat him or her, no real idea what to say. They went home with their anxiety intact, as well as their old fears and their new shame, walked around on eggshells for a few days and within a short time found themselves back in the cycle of heartache which had taken them to the hospital in the first place.

Many psychiatric hospitals have been closed down over the past twenty years, as governments have moved psychiatric patients into community houses. Seriously ill patients have become the responsibility of mental health units in public hospitals, but there they have to compete for medical attention with people critically ill with injuries and physical illness. Nor are these hospitals geared for the long stays involved in mental health treatments.

Writing in *The Australian* newspaper in January, 1997, Sydney psychiatrist Dr Jean Lennane pointed out that national policy split drug and alcohol services from mental health ten years ago, despite more than fifty percent of young people with a serious mental illness also having difficulties with alcohol and marijuana.

'It [the national health policy] abolished any longer-term in-patient treatment for alcohol and drug problems and in rigidly adopting a harm-minimisation policy, has made abstinence [from drugs and alcohol] a dirty word, even for young children,' said Dr Lennane.

The main problem facing harassed and overworked public hospital casualty staff is knowing where to put young men and women who are a danger to themselves, particularly when they usually reach crisis point late at night or during the weekend. The practical problem of deciding what to do with them is complicated by the general bias against young people who are frequently regarded as attention-seeking, manipulative and difficult.

All states and territories are currently in the process of revising their Mental Health Acts to pull them into line with the United Nations recommendations on mental health. New protocols and policies are being developed to ensure that young people are not as neglected and discriminated against as they have been in the past and that families are more involved where possible.

Current mental health laws give hospital doctors the authority to place a person into hospital if they are mentally ill and constitute a danger to themselves *or* if they are experiencing a mental health crisis which has rendered them temporarily out of control of their actions. This type of involuntary hospital admission is known as being scheduled.

Understanding the current mental health system is difficult as the procedures involved in the treatment of involuntary admissions vary a great deal, not only from state to state but from hospital to hospital.

Doctors are obliged by law to use the least restrictive alternative when treating mental health patients. If they believe it is in the patient's best interest to remain in hospital for longer than a few (usually three) working days, the case must go before a magistrate, who has to approve the extended stay after examining the medical evidence concerning the patient's condition.

When a young person has attempted suicide, or if a doctor thinks they are at risk of suicide, involuntary admission and treatment is usually recommended. Ideally, this involves keeping the patient in hospital for an assessment by the hospital psychiatrist or social worker, who then devises a treatment plan, usually involving antidepressant medication and counselling.

Unfortunately, unless there is a diagnosis of acute psychiatric illness, the serious shortage of beds in most hospitals discourages mental health admissions, particularly at weekends or at night. Doctors are generally unwilling to schedule young people whose problems are obviously related to alcohol and drug dependence. An adolescent who has made a suicide attempt is more likely to be treated for physical injuries or overdose damage, given a prescription for antidepressants, handed a card containing the telephone number of a counselling service and sent home – if he or she has a home to go to.

There is rarely much follow-up. Finding counselling or getting further treatment is up to the patient or the family. 'How could we be expected to chase them all up?' asked one hospital doctor. 'By the middle of the next week we've seen another twenty or thirty people who all need urgent treatment. We just don't have the time or the resources to help them if they won't help themselves.'

The provision of time and human kindness would be a huge step forward in the prevention of youth suicide.

According to Barry Taylor, the real tragedy of youth suicide is that those who do complete a suicide after several previous attempts are often the victims of a system which is not geared to long-term counselling. 'After ten days they've usually been processed and they're out.' Girls are more likely than boys to come into the hospital system with self-inflicted injuries. 'Boys who are as despairing as these girls have usually been placed in the Juvenile Justice system by this age. Young men are much more likely to take out their despair and rage in crime than young women.'

The girls appear most frequently on a busy Saturday night, when the stretched and harassed young registrar on duty is required to tick an appropriate box so that each case can be duly processed.

'They have to decide whether this is this self-harming behaviour or attempted suicide,' said Barry. 'But if this girl has slashed her wrists, what is she really saying? Is it: "I feel like shit. My body looks like shit. By slashing my wrists I am letting out the pain. It is oozing out with the blood" ... Or does she mean: "Hey, I'm feeling absolutely miserable. There's nobody I can tell, no one is interested in how I feel ... but look, look at me. My hands are cut. My wrists are bleeding. Take notice of me; I've hurt myself"?'

Girls who make genuine suicide attempts don't usually want to die; they are just wondering whether they want to live. 'They keep turning up in our hospitals and they often have histories of chronic abuse,' said Barry. 'They are mentally ill, but not all the time. When they are well they worry themselves sick about what will happen next time they get depressed. The trouble is that when they are being treated for mental illness, they feel isolated; we take away their peer supports who are so important to them.'

But some of them recover. Just as a catalyst may push young men and women into suicide, a new development may pull them back into life. 'At twenty-two or twenty-three, some of them seem to mature, almost overnight,' said Barry. 'A good relationship, a job, the birth of a child – something happens that persuades them to start the hard work of building a life.'

A thirteen-year-old girl who had lost her friend through suicide a few weeks previously approached a youth worker and said she was frightened; she thought she might want to end it all. The youth worker took her to a hospital where they waited for five hours for someone to help her. The doctor on duty was advised to prescribe her some antidepressants and send her home. This is not what she wanted. She wanted somebody to help her, to look after her. There was nobody. The doctor said to her: 'You're not going to kill yourself, are you? Because if you are I'm going to have to lock you up.'

'They don't need hospitals or doctors or pills,' said Barry Taylor. 'They need support. They need someone to care.'

ADAM

Adam Kemp completed suicide in January, 1996. Since his death – between periods of raw grief and deep depression, and often against her own better judgement – his mother, Ruth Anderson, has become involved in the drive to reduce youth suicide deaths. At times, she asks with anguish how she can possibly advise anyone else when she feels she herself failed her son. But as the figures climb – eight young people in her area alone died in 1996 – she is overwhelmed with the need to take action.

While Ruth Anderson's respect for Adam's intensely private nature has prevented her from giving intimate details of his life, her practical and realistic suggestions for improvements in the health system could provide effective tools in the construction of a program to slow the youth suicide epidemic. She has been invited by the Premier of New South Wales to present her recommendations to the House of Representatives in the NSW Government.

'My son, Adam, was a tall, lean, good looking, strong-featured young man, who had achieved a great deal in his short life and had a future full of promise. A good scholar until the age of seventeen, when he chose to leave school early, a gifted musician and a brilliant sportsman, he had won a golfing scholarship just before his death. Respected by his peers, he was a precise, quiet and private person; I've been told by others that he was an asset to our small community. His death, alone and in the dark, has left a void in the lives of many.

'A baby, a boy, a man – nineteen years has gone too fast. But then, Adam lived fast. Everything had to happen yesterday and every hour had to be filled. He must have known his journey here would be short.

'For most of his first ten years as an only child, Adam had my undivided attention and also that of his devoted grandmother. When after six years into my second marriage I had two more children, the fact that he became angry and jealous I put down to the overload of love he had initially experienced. As he matured during adolescence, I felt he needed to learn to be confident in his own ability to control his life; after all, he had behaved very independently from an early age.

'I recognise now that during a period when he really craved some restraints, I was loosening the reins. Young people seem ever keen to separate from parental supervision but they still want to know that you care about them. Adam became so removed and adamant that he was his own person and didn't need me that I didn't insist; I neglected to make this vital contribution to his life.

'I observed serious changes in Adam for three or four months before his first attempt on his life but I attributed them to external circumstances over which I had no control. He had become increasingly irritable and uncooperative, he skipped meals, ate poorly and his sleep pattern appeared insufficient for the intense levels of energy on which he was functioning. Personal hygiene took a back seat and he seemed angry and frustrated with where he was in his life. I supposed all these changes were consistent with a difficult adolescence. I was so wrong.

'In October, 1995, we had a futile argument during which I had tried to show him what damage his lifestyle – the stress of changing from one job to another which involved shift work, erratic meals, little sleep and hours and hours shut up in his room with his computer – was doing to his health.

Later that day I returned home to find he had taken an overdose of tablets.

'We arrived at the accident and emergency ward of the local hospital in the middle of the evening. He was given treatment to eliminate the drug. The nursing staff were gentle, although their attitude seemed to be: "Well, here's another one". Throughout the night, Adam wafted in and out of consciousness, interspersed with regular trips to the lavatory as his body was purged of the poison in his system.

'In the morning a woman from the local psychiatric hospital came to see him. She was accusatory and judgmental. She asked him: "Did you think how you would upset your mother?" She talked at him rather than counselling him, although he was so drowsy I imagine anything she said fell on deaf ears.

'Adam was not an habitual attempter. He was an eighteen-year-old in despair. I would have appreciated more care and empathy, leading to an offer of support in answer to his obvious cry for help. She even laughed when I asked if he would be able to drive later that day, assuring me that the drug would be out of his system by then. It seemed unimportant that he *had* made an attempt on his life, had his stomach pumped and spent the night in hospital under observation. I am obviously ignorant of the protocol in place to deal with these situations but I question its effectiveness when such a negative and flippant attitude is expressed to a person in pain.

'We were referred to a psychologist but seeing him proved to be a very negative experience for Adam, who said he wanted to forget the whole thing and get on with his life. Both the mental health worker and the psychologist assured me I would be contacted and I was told I could expect a visit from the local youth centre. In the following days and weeks, however, I heard from none of these people.

'I was confused as to how and where to find help. The institutional therapy seemed extreme. As nobody followed up Adam's attempt on his life, I felt that they must have considered this unnecessary and wondered if I was over-reacting.

'Neither of these two health professionals gave me guidelines about the "after-care" of someone who had attempted suicide. Neither advised me about risks or signs of crisis, or strategies to employ in order to prevent another attempt. Neither suggested antidepressant therapy, which may have assisted him to return to a receptive and rational level.

'I have recently discovered that many suicide prevention services exist in the community. It saddens me that we were not referred to any of them. Our confusion and helplessness simply increased over the following weeks.

'Three months later Adam made a second attempt on his life. This time his act was complete and final.

'I now live with the guilt I feel for not somehow relieving Adam's hurt. This is my worst parental failure. I was unable to relieve my son's pain. My punishment will be life long.

'Since Adam's death, as the rate of suicide in my area has increased drastically, I have become convinced that the area of suicide care needs drastic revision. Many of the health workers to whom I have spoken have felt exasperated and frustrated by the current system. If Adam had been an asthmatic in respiratory distress, a diabetic in a coma or an epileptic in a seizure, his health care would have been monitored until it was established that he was on an upward curve to improvement. Why is mental health less important, when according to a prediction by the World Health Organization, by the year 2020, depression will be the main cause of death and disability in the world?

'I would like to see unification and solidarity among the providers of health services in our community. I would like to see egos left at the door while people work together to achieve the common objective of saving lives. I would like to see a more responsible media playing a crucial role in helping young people help each other rather than taking a voyeuristic interest in the more gruesome details some reporters glean from sitting in on the inquests.

'With other survivors of suicide I have been asked to make some recommendations to the New South Wales House of Representatives. If some changes can be implemented to educate the community about suicide awareness and prevention, to improve the response of the health profession to people in crisis and to ease the pain of those bereaved by suicide, then the loss I share with so many others will possess an element of reason.

'Most of the suggestions below are relevant to my personal situation and could perhaps have made a difference to the outcome. I will never know.

'My recommendations include:

- A national education program to teach the public how to recognise depression and its negative effects on us, our jobs, our families and our communities, including *a central phone number* which connects a person to the service he or she needs.

- Sympathetic coverage in the media of such issues as depression in all age groups, sexuality – including support and safety in "coming out" for both young people and their parents, unemployment, domestic violence and relationship breakdowns.

- Effective suicide intervention procedures at hospitals. Policies and procedures should be established to manage attempted and completed suicide with unprejudiced and non-judgmental staff. Scaring people away doesn't fix the problem. Prompt and consistent follow-up should be an essential part of these procedures.

- The education of *young people* in the life skills they need to cope with loss and change while maintaining self-esteem and self-respect.
- The education of *parents* about appropriate ways of responding to their adolescents' needs in these vitally important years.
- The education of *general practitioners* in how to recognise depression in young people and how to teach them about using antidepressant medication when required.
- The education of young people about getting help when depression and despair never seem to lift. The youth media could play an important part in this.
- The establishment of a crisis centre for youth, run by people trained in counselling and situated in an area central to the local community. Early detection of a problem means early intervention and prevention of tragedy.
- The appointment of a child and adolescent psychiatrist or at best, more psychologists, in each local community – and the advertising of this service so that people in trouble know there is someone to whom they can turn for help.
- The appointment of a protector or mentor for the health workers themselves, to relieve and support them in their stressful work.
- For the families of people who have attempted or completed suicide, a trained counsellor from the hospital or local suicide support group, to be available on a twenty-four hour roster, for support and guidance in the hours when you feel too numb or shocked to know what to do.
- In the aftermath of suicide, a "parcel of hope" for the bereaved, to be issued by the attending police chaplain, counsellor or local suicide support representative. The parcel could contain:
  - ♣ police – ID card and phone number
  - ♣ coroner – name, phone number and office hours

+ morgue – phone number and contact name to arrange "goodbye" visit, plus an outline of what to expect and the pros and cons of such a visit
+ counsellors – names, addresses and phone numbers of people trained in bereavement support
+ checklist of things which must be done almost immediately – police statement, contact with coroner, funeral arrangements, appropriate responses to calls
+ a copy of *Surviving the Pain* published by Rose Education
+ a copy of *After Suicide: Help for the Bereaved* (published by Hill of Content) by Dr Sheila Clark
+ a copy of *Let's Live* newsletter from Suicide Prevention Australia which contains a further reading list and local suicide support group addresses and contact numbers plus relevant and sensitive articles.

'Above all, we need community awareness concerning the problem of youth suicide and what to do about it. Other national campaigns have been successful in saving lives – there's the road safety programs, Sudden Infant Death Syndrome, even Clean Up Australia. What about a Care and Repair program? While we have become a disposable society, I don't believe that life should fall into that category.

'Our community is hurting. Resources have been pushed to the limit. We don't need further cuts, we need expanded resources, sustained and advanced funds. For us surviving parents, this grief is ever after. The isolation, guilt, despair and frustration that most of us feel is the legacy our children have left us. Now, too late, we understand what they must have been going through in the days and hours leading up to their death.

'It would be naive to believe that we can make suicide go away, but with care, intelligence, knowledge, sensitivity and genuine concern for our fellow man, perhaps we could hope to reduce these frightening figures.

'We have to start somewhere. No one should have to farewell their child at a morgue.'

JAAKKO: A MATE

JAAKKO: 'I reckon the police picked on Collin a bit too much. He would be cruising in his HR – it was a beautiful car. It was his pride and joy and he had built it up from scratch; it really stood out. Police don't know anything about a car like that. They were always defecting him – his racing shift, his tyres. It wasn't all that loud; it wasn't as loud as a train or a plane.

'None of us drank much. We were too busy working on our cars. Collin would be at it until one or two in the morning. We weren't interested in going to the pubs and clubs.

'He and Sharon used to fight a bit but no more than anybody else – no more than Lindy and me. Everyone was having their ups and downs.

'The trouble with Collin was he would clam up. He kept a lot inside. Once he told me his parents were getting into all this religious stuff. I said: "Why not go with them and have a look?" I would. I poke my head in everywhere to see what goes on in life – you can always learn something. But Collin wouldn't. Going to something like that with his parents wouldn't be cool.

'Collin bought a boat and a whole crowd of us used to go water skiing. Collin really liked his young brother, Adam. He used to say: "Let's go and get Adam and take him out on the boat".

'When he came around and asked if he could move into the spare room at our place I had no objection at all. I'd do anything to help a mate and Collin was one of the two best friends I have ever had.

'I borrowed my brother's truck and we went and got his stuff. He was unhappy with his parents. He said they didn't like him having the car. When they had visitors they'd say: "Collin built this himself", but afterwards they would be at him to get rid of it.

'So he came to live with us. He had started drinking a bit by then, although not all the time. When things didn't go sweet for Collin he drank and he had troubles with alcohol because it made him depressed. It made him violent.

'Like when he had trouble with the tow truck. He wanted to be a tow truck driver and he was really stoked about getting this job because he hadn't worked for a while. But the truck they gave him was a real bomb.

'The radiator hose blew. The bull bar fell off. Then it broke down on the expressway. The hand brake didn't work so one day the truck rolled over someone's garden. He put the HR on it and his front guard was damaged. He'd get real cranky and he'd have a drink.

'I realised his problems were really serious the night he tried to gas himself. When I got home I found the back door had been kicked in. I suppose he couldn't find his key.

'There was more damage done in the lounge room, although he hadn't broken any of our stuff, just his own. I went into the garage and saw what he'd been doing. I found Collin in his room, in bed. He was real crook.

'I tried to talk some sense into him. I said: "Look, Collin, I know times are tough and that, but there are a lot of other times to come up. I'm doing it tough too, I've run out of work and I've had to sell my ski boat. I know it's hard getting money together. But if you do this you'll end up in the worse place you'll ever be." I'm a little bit religious and I told him straight out that it just wasn't worth it. "Things will start to sweeten up later on, you know," I said. "Everyone goes through a hard time."

'He seemed all right. He seemed to understand what I was getting at, once the grog wore off.

'I saw his dad later that day, when he wanted Collin to have a look at his new car. I didn't tell him about Collin trying to kill himself. I thought it was a freak thing – he wasn't likely to do it again. He was pretty drunk, after all. I thought I had talked some sense into him. Anyway, he wasn't real happy with his parents at the time and I wasn't sure whether I should say anything.

'I don't think he was taking drugs. I don't use marijuana and I wouldn't let anyone smoke it in my house. He was having hassles with this other bloke we both knew; it was over a girl. The guy wanted to fight him. I don't know why Collin didn't just have it out with him instead of turning his back. Collin was real fit from skiing and going to the gym. He would have given him a good run for his money but he didn't have enough confidence in himself. They would have been better off having a scuffle and getting it out of their systems. But after Collin tried to gas himself I told this bloke to lay off him. I told him it wasn't nice when a mate was so depressed. The bloke didn't care.

'A while after that Collin moved back to his parents' house and I went off to work in Katoomba for a while. When I came back one weekend I met Collin at the pub and we were real happy to see each other. We were just two walking grins. We sent the girls off inside to the disco and we talked for a couple of hours, catching up on everything. Collin was great to have a yarn to. I have to admit that when he was living with us he would get on edge and have a bit of a snap and I would clam up because I didn't want to hassle him while he was depressed. But that paid off because we were still mates.

'When we went inside to find the girls again, Collin and Sharon told me they were thinking of getting married. They asked me if I wanted to be the best man. I said: "Oh yeah!

No worries". Straight away I thought things had to be going better for him.

'Two weeks later I came home from Katoomba again and I was real excited because I'd saved enough money to buy a quad racer. That's a sort of motorbike with four wheels, and Collin got me interested in them because he had one of his own. You race them in the sand dunes. They are heaps of fun. Lindy and I drove past the hotel and I knew they were all in there because it was a Friday night. I thought of going in and telling Collin I was getting the quad racer. But I'm not much into pubs and that so we drove on past. I decided I'd go around on Saturday and tell him all about it.

'That was Friday night, November 13th.'

PART THREE

COLLIN: NOVEMBER 14

Collin and Sharon drove away down the dusty road from his parents' house and waved to Jan, who was just arriving home from a walk. They took Sharon's car. Collin's HR, gleaming in the late-afternoon sunshine, was parked in the driveway at the side of the house.

It was early, so they dropped in to see a friend who lived nearby. They had a few drinks and smoked some marijuana. Next they called in at a party where Collin and a mate shared a bottle of Southern Comfort.

It was close to midnight when they arrived at the hotel, where they met more of their friends. Sharon felt excited, happy, a little high. With Cathy's wedding only a week away, marriage plans dominated the conversation. Maybe she and Collin would be the next couple to tie the knot ...

The guy, when he loomed towards them in the smoky bar, was familiar. He threatened Collin. He had done it before. He was one of the minority of people (along with some local policemen) who did not like Collin Schultz. Sharon can't remember why.

'They were both full of alcohol,' she said. 'Collin wouldn't back down if someone threw a punch at him but he was too smart to start anything. He walked outside. He was horribly angry.

'I tried to calm him down, but he told me to go back inside. He wanted to go home on his own, he said. He was going to walk all the way from Ourimbah – about eight kilometres.

He went off into the darkness, heading up to the road, and he was so cranky he kicked a car on the way. He kicked it so hard I was surprised his leg didn't snap.

'Then he started to run.'

Most Saturdays Ron rose early to go running with his mates from Trotters, a running club. He often met Collin, who would be just arriving home. On this particular Saturday in November, Collin's car, the beautiful old blue and white Holden, was already at home.

It was in the way. Ron had borrowed a trailer to get wood chips for the front and back garden. Collin's car was blocking the access to the back yard. When Ron returned from his run and went to collect the trailer, he realised he wouldn't be able to get to the job in hand until Collin moved his car.

Deciding he could wait until his son arrived home, Ron left the trailer out the front and started work on the garden. They had only been in the house a few months and there was a lot to do. He dug, snipped, pruned and weeded around the new shrubs – but he had planned to use that trailer before the spring sunshine became too hot and not for the first time, he cursed his son's pride and joy.

Fourteen-year-old Adam gave the HR an admiring glance as he and a friend who had slept over collected their bikes and set off for a ride. One day Adam planned to have a car just like his brother's.

Julianne woke up in a panic from the worst dream she had ever had. 'Collin was calling to me from a dark place,' she told Jan. She was almost in tears. 'It was like some sort of gaol, and I was climbing up steps, trying to find him, but I couldn't. He was calling my name but I couldn't get to him.'

'Gaol?' said Jan sardonically. 'Well that's highly on the cards.' But she hugged her daughter and suggested a trip to

Sydney to take her mind off her troubles. She offered to take Julianne's boyfriend, Robbie, as well. They could all do a bit of last minute wedding shopping. For Jan, such a spur of the moment decision was unusual. They came out of the house and left in Jan's car, forgetting to mention to Ron how far they were going, and why.

Ron finished everything he could do in the front garden. There was still no sign of Collin. He gave up and walked down the back yard to get the wheelbarrow from the shed.

'I pulled up the roller door and I looked in. Collin was there. I thought: "Well *here* you are. What are you doing in here?" I don't think I actually got around to saying anything out loud. But that's what I thought when I first saw him.

'Collin had a grin on his face and he seemed to be just standing there, because his boots had slipped down his feet a bit. Then I saw the rope.

'For a fleeting second I thought: "You bastard." I thought he was playing a trick on me. Then I said: "No". And I started to scream.'

As his mind swelled with pain, Ron fell silent. After a few interminable seconds of utter horror and helplessness, he looked around for the set of steps he needed to reach the rafter. He cut through the rope with a file and the weight of his son fell upon him. They crashed to the ground together.

Ron lay on the ground with the body of his son across his own. He struggled to his feet and looked down at Collin's face.

'I had always said suicide was a cowardly act,' said Ron slowly. His voice shuddered; he paused for a while and then continued. 'But I realised that all the pain and suffering Collin must have had inside had become too much for him. Nobody could do that to themselves unless their life had become just too hard to bear. I said to him: "I understand". And I forgave my son for what he had done.'

Neighbours who had heard Ron screaming were gathering hesitantly at the edge of the yard. He left the shed, carefully closing the door, straightened up, told them he was fine. He went into the house and dialled triple 0.

The police came with an ambulance and Ron took them down to the shed. When he went back to the house the phone was ringing. It was Sharon, asking to speak to Collin.

'No,' replied Ron. 'Things are bad.' He hung up.

Sharon put down the phone and was filled with an awful sense of foreboding. She rang a couple of friends to see if they had heard if something had happened to Collin. They hadn't. She thought of Collin running up the hill, disappearing into the dark. He was going home, he said. He must have gone home. Ron hadn't said whether he was home or not.

She rang a close friend and asked him to go around to the Schultz house to find out what was going on. He brought her the bad news an hour later.

Adam saw the police car and the ambulance outside his house and came to investigate. Ron told him what had happened and he went into his room. 'One of the policemen asked me if I wanted to go and stay with Adam for a while but I said no. I knew there were official things to be done. Typical of me, wasn't it? Thinking I was doing the correct thing instead of going to my boy.' A little while later, one of the police came into the living room and said: 'Your young chap has jumped out of his bedroom window and is racing away up the hill'.

Ron ran outside. The neighbours pointed the way Adam had gone and his father ran after him and eventually found him sitting alone on a rock in the scrub. 'Come home,' he pleaded but Adam refused. 'I don't want to come home, Dad,' he said. 'I'll be okay.'

'Please,' Ron begged. 'Please come home with me.'

They were back when Jan, Julianne and Robbie arrived home from their shopping trip at 3 p.m. Ron met them at the door and told Julianne and Robbie to go up the street to buy some bread and milk. He wanted to tell Jan first. A counsellor from the local hospital was waiting in the house.

'He let me bring all the groceries in,' said Jan, 'and then he took me into the bedroom and told me that Collin had hung himself in the shed.'

Jan shook her head over and over again. 'I don't believe you,' she said. 'I'm not listening to this. I won't believe it.'

But she knew straight away that it was true.

Collin was dead. Collin, with his wonderful smile. Collin, her beautiful baby boy, who always cuddled close. Collin, her soft, hard, courageous, cowardly, fast, slow, speed-crazy, car-loving son, had killed himself. In the shed.

How could he do that? How could he do that to himself? How could he do that to her?

A lead-like heaviness settled in her stomach and stayed there.

How could he do it to the family?

'Where's Adam?' Jan asked suddenly. 'What about Julianne?' A new horror sank claws into her heart. In such a small community, somebody else might be telling Julianne right at that moment, that her brother was dead. She asked Ron if Sharon knew what had happened.

Julianne and Robbie came back. Despite her dream, Julianne assumed her father had sent her away because he was preparing some sort of nice surprise. Her parents told her and Robbie the truth.

People kept arriving at the house. Friends. Collin's boss. Neighbours. Runners. Sharon, supported by two girlfriends.

'An hour or so after we came home,' said Jan, 'I remembered the wedding. "What about the wedding?" I said.

"What about the wedding?"' It was one week away. People were coming from everywhere. Cathy would have to make a decision about the wedding but Cathy couldn't be contacted. She was at her flat in Sydney but she wasn't answering her phone. 'She wasn't home,' said Jan bleakly.

About three o'clock a mate dropped in on Jaakko and Lindy. 'Have you heard what Collin's done?' he asked. Jaakko was exasperated. 'What's he done *now*?'

Cathy, her fiance Dean and some friends had driven to a park near Windsor for the day. When they arrived back at their Sydney flat that evening, her father and her younger brother were waiting outside in the car. Ron asked Cathy if they could have a cup of tea and they all went inside.

'It takes such a long time before you realise someone is really dead,' said Cathy. 'It's not like the ads for car accidents that you see on the television, where they understand straight away. I went and threw up but I still didn't believe it had happened.

'I didn't want to go home. I knew once I got there, that would make it real.'

Ron arrived back home without her. Jan could not conceive that her eldest child would not want to be with her family at such a time. She rang Cathy and asked her why she hadn't come. 'I thought you wouldn't want Dean there,' said Cathy. But they told her they wanted them both and a few hours later the whole family was together again. All but one.

'We didn't sleep much that night,' said Ron.

'It just got worse and worse from then on,' said Jan.

The day after Collin died, ADAM SCHULTZ, then fourteen, wrote and illustrated his own record of his brother's life.

A Book of the Best Brother in the World: Collin Jeffrey Schultz.

Collin was born 16th September, 1969.

He was born at Ryde Hospital, Sydney.

He lived a happy twenty-three years and two months of working on bikes and cars and boats. Collin worked at many different places but by far liked working the most up at Newcastle Repco as a mechanic. He died 14th November 1992.

Collin's death was a quick one. He hung himself in the shed. Collin had thought about it sometimes but he had never discussed it with anyone. He did it where he felt comfortable which was at home in the backyard. Collin knew Dad was the strong one and I think Collin wanted Dad to find him and that's what happened.

I just hope Collin knows how many people there are down here who love him.

I have always liked Dad and Collin the most out of the family. I think Collin is the best brother anyone in the world could have. Everything Collin did with me or every place Collin would take me, I liked.

When I was about ten or eleven years old Collin lived down the street from us and I used to ride my pushbike down there, just to see him and talk to him. I loved my brother.

Habits: Collin never really had any bad habits. He was never a person who was addicted to alcohol, he drank a little bit but that was it. I remember once when I was at a party with him, everyone was drinking and he had a beer in his hand. When Collin thought no one was looking he tipped half of it out, but I saw him do it.

He doesn't smoke or have any tattoos although there was a time when Collin wanted this particular tattoo. I don't think God wanted him to have that tattoo or any of them because there was only one person who could do that tattoo and every time Collin would go down there that person would not be there or Collin would not have enough money. He just wasn't made for a tattoo.

There are a few things that Collin is addicted to and one of them is fixing up cars. Another thing is Coca Cola.

Collin taught me how to ride a bike. He used to hold on to the seat and walk behind me while I pedalled and steered. I always told him don't let go, don't let go but then I'd be riding along and I'd turn the bike around and I'd see Collin right up the end of the street.

Collin taught me everything there is to know about a bike. He knew it all by the age of eight years old.

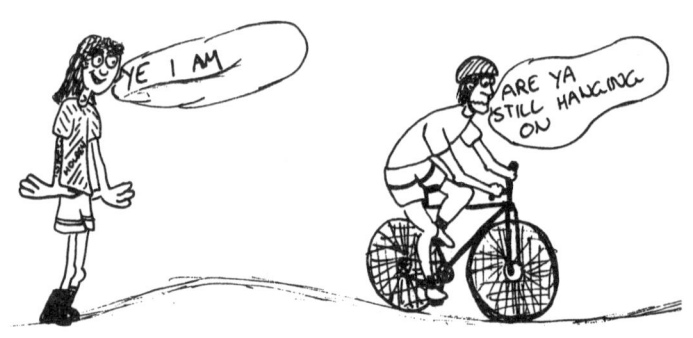

I loved it when we would wrestle or muck around. Sometimes he used to hurt me but I never told him because I didn't want him to stop. I really liked it.

Just before the accident he asked me if I would teach him some karate. I was so happy and looking forward to it so much and now I can't do that.

Collin built himself a very nice HR Holden 308 V8 stroker, Peter Brock blue with a good interior. It had a nine inch diff and a few parts of a chevy thrown in here and there.

I was the only person who he ever let wash it. He trusted me and I will always remember that.

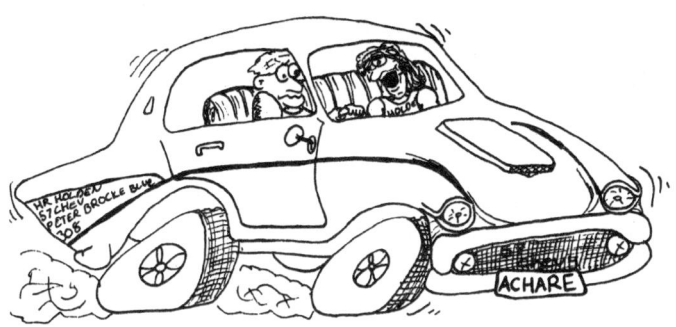

Collin's speed boat was one of the only things that would get him away from his cars. One of the things Collin did for me with his boat was to teach me how to ski. Collin could go on one ski. He used to do three-sixties (that's a full circle) on a kneeboard.

The Thrill of Speed: I think Collin enjoyed things that went fast. As a kid, whenever you went to a fun park or a festival he would race off to the dodgem cars or the go-carts. Now he has grown up he likes cars. When he was about twenty-one years old he started liking boats but not just any old tugboat. It had to be a speedboat.

He has been talking a lot lately about getting a Harley Davidson.

1992 was a good year for Collin. I think he was the happiest he has been for a long time. Sharon was a great help for Collin. She loved him just as much as Jan, Ron, Cathy, Julianne and Adam – that's me. Collin said that he was thinking about marrying Sharon in 1993. Jaakko was going to be the best man. Cathy met Dean in 1991 and is marrying him this year, this weekend to be exact. Julianne is going out with Robbie and I think she wants to marry him but I don't know yet.

Collin's funeral is this Wednesday.

Julianne, Cathy, Ron, Jan and Sharon went to see Collin before the funeral. 'It wasn't him,' said Jan. 'They didn't have the hair right. It just didn't look like him at all.'

Because Collin wasn't religious the funeral service was held at Palmdale Lawn Cemetery.

The following March there was an inquest. Alcohol, marijuana and amphetamines had been found in Collin's system. While none of the drugs were present in excessive amounts, they formed a mix which was described by the coroner as a cocktail waiting to explode, particularly in a person with Collin's personality.

'Looking back,' said Jan, 'I realised his paranoia about being hunted down by the police was probably caused by the drugs. We had no idea about the drugs.'

Ron initially blamed himself entirely for Collin's death. 'But at least he came home and did it here,' he said. 'That was the nicest thing he could have done under the circumstances. He must have thought: "Dad will find me. Dad will know what to do". I am not angry with him at all.'

But Jan wanted to scream at her son. What would have happened if Adam had gone to the shed that morning? Or the friend who was sleeping over? What about his sister's wedding in one week's time? What about Julianne's birthday in a fortnight? What about the future? How could they all go on living, if Collin was dead?

'Look what you have done to this family!' she raged at him. 'This was a great family! Now everything has changed!'

JASON: JULY 9

Jason drove down the mountain to see his family on Friday night. He wanted to talk to Lee and Peter about the girls. They were surprised – normally when he thought Ceane and Charmaine were getting themselves into strife, he would speak to them without letting his mother and father know. He saw himself as the buffer between his parents and the relationship disasters which entangled and sometimes endangered his sisters.

'Jason's way,' said Lee, 'was to give them an ear bashing and tell them to sort themselves out.'

But on that Friday he came straight to his parents. He was seriously concerned about Ceane and Charmaine and he wanted Peter and Lee to take control. He told them he was also worried about Kurt. He had discovered that his fifteen-year-old brother was smoking marijuana and while it might have sounded like a case of the pot and the kettle, he just didn't think it was a good idea any more.

Before they came to any conclusions the phone rang. Lee was called out to an emergency. She left Jason with his father, still talking. He left eventually, with the promise that he would return on Sunday to take young Keiran to the big football match in Sydney.

On the following night Jason rang Lee and told her he wouldn't be able to make it on Sunday after all. Knowing how disappointed Keiran was going to be, Lee asked him if he needed money for the trip. Jason said no, he just couldn't make it.

Late on Sunday afternoon, Jason rang his mate Joel. 'We talked about Manly beating Parramatta and he sounded a bit down but I didn't pay much attention.' About 7 p.m. Jason rang Mark, the second of his three closest friends.

'We just talked for a bit and then he told me to look after myself because he was going away for a while,' said Mark. 'I tried to find out where he was heading but he wouldn't say. Then I asked what he was going to do with his furniture and he said he wouldn't be needing it. That sounded a bit strange, and I remembered that he'd been giving quite a bit of his other stuff away.'(Jason took extremely good care of his skin. After days of dirty work on the lines he used creams and lotions to remove the ingrained dirt from his pores. Giving no reason, he had given his cleansing creams away to his mates' girlfriends.)

Finally Mark said: 'Well, give me a ring when you get there.'

'Mate,' said Jason, 'where I'm going there are no phones.'

'That's when I realised what he was going to do,' said Mark, who immediately hung up the phone, raced out of his house, and drove out of town and up the mountain to the little town of Bracken.

As he pulled up outside, he saw his friend sitting in his car in the driveway of his house, talking into his mobile phone, and weeping. He was making a third call, this time to Jack, the boy who kept them laughing with his witty cartoons. Jack too, suddenly guessed the truth. He tried to keep Jason talking for a while but finally hung up. He leapt into his car and headed up the mountain.

Mark approached Jason's car and yelled at him through the driver's window. 'He wouldn't get out. He sounded all dopey and slow, but he was very strong, very determined. I tried to talk to him. I tried to stop him. He said it was half-done anyway and I shouldn't stop him. Then he gunned the motor and drove out into the street. He did this massive U-turn and drove off.

'I didn't realise what he was already doing until I saw the back of the car, and the hose in the exhaust. I got back in my own car then and tried to chase him but I lost him. I was in a panic. I drove to the police station and reported what was happening. Then I went back to Jason's and Jack was there.'

Jack kept watch at Jason's house, in case he came back. Mark drove back to town and picked up Joel. 'Jason's place was immaculate but he had trashed his kitchen,' said Joel. 'He had smashed the microwave and broken a table and there were broken cups everywhere. We thought he must have had a brain snap.' The three friends went together in search of Jason. They couldn't understand how their funny mate, the bloke who had always kept them laughing, had fallen so low. He'd had a few problems in the past few weeks, but hadn't they all? Surely there was no way he would go through with this craziness, surely not ... ?

'We drove all round the mountains,' said Mark. 'We went to all his little favourite hiding spots, all the places he'd found for himself over the years when he wanted to go off and be on his own. We couldn't find him anywhere.'

When they ran out of places to look they drove back down into the town. Mark and Joel dropped Jack off at his home; they had decided Lee and Peter should be told what was going on. Jack made the call while the other two went to the police station to see if there was any news of their friend.

Jack rang Peter and Lee and asked if Jason had been around or in touch with them.

'No, Jack, not today,' Lee replied. 'What's wrong?' Jack wanted to tell his mate's mum that there was nothing wrong, nothing at all. Instead he told her the truth.

Lee put down the phone and her great big heart turned over. No. It wasn't possible. Not Jason, of all people. Jason was her rock. Jason had never caused any trouble.

The boys had to be wrong.

Her mind was sluggish. Nothing made sense. She decided to go to the police station to see if there had been any accidents. She couldn't face going alone, so she drove to Charmaine's flat to see if she could come with her. Peter said he would stay with the children. He watched Lee drive away, sat down and waited for the phone to ring again.

Ceane was at home alone in her flat. She fell asleep with her clothes on and dreamed she was at a funeral. She had no idea who was in the coffin and woke up convinced that something had happened to her boyfriend, who hadn't come home. Someone was knocking at the door.

Her sister Charmaine was standing outside in the dark. 'They think Jason's going to kill himself,' she said.

Jason was found in his car, on a lonely mountain road with a spectacular view. In a house not far away, guests at a dinner party had noticed his car. One of the visitors, a male nurse, tried to revive him. The ambulance was called and Jason was taken down the mountains to the local hospital.

Lee, Ceane and Charmaine drove to the police station. With every turn of the wheel, Lee's heart pumped more loudly than the engine. No. Not her boy, this special boy. The one she planned. The one she kept. Not Jason, the first delicate link in the chain of love she had been clasping around herself for twenty-four years.

Five minutes after Mark and Joel reached the police station, a report came in from the Bracken police saying that Jason had been found and that he was no longer living. The police asked the boys if they would prefer to tell Jason's parents themselves.

The night was dark and very cold.

Lee and her two older daughters arrived at the police station just before midnight. The moon had slipped out of sight. Ceane and Charmaine saw Jason's two friends come out of the building and walk towards their car. Lee went to meet them.

'They told Mum what Jason had done,' sobbed Ceane. 'She let out this huge cry. It was this awful mother-cry of pain.'

Lee's howl of anguish echoed up into the mountain and filled what was left of the night.

The police came to the house and told Peter, who began to weep. The kids all woke up. 'I just knew,' said Stacey softly. 'Dad didn't have to tell me.'

The police drove to the Connor house with Lee and picked up Peter. They were then taken down to the big town at the foot of the mountains. There, in the morgue, they identified the body of their son, Jason, who had died from carbon monoxide poisoning at the age of twenty-four.

'Telling Mrs Connor was the hardest thing I have ever had to do in my life,' said Joel. Nearly two years later, the tears sting the young man's eyes. 'I felt so helpless. We could have stopped him. By phoning us he was reaching out for help, but we couldn't find him. We didn't get to him in time.

'His favourite American football jacket that a mate had brought him back from Hawaii was folded neatly, with his hat, on the seat beside him. His seat was tipped back. He was just lying there, waiting to be taken. But why? Why? You keep asking yourself why and you start to think you're getting somewhere with it and then you find you are back at the same place.'

Kurt was away at a cadets camp. They sent him home and he arrived not knowing which of his two brothers had died.

'It was if he had planned it,' said Peter. 'In the kitchen the microwave was smashed, but everything else was in order. Look at this place – there's nothing in order here, it's a lived-in house. But his house was bloody spotless, not a speck of dirt or dust. His clothes were clean and neatly folded. He had paid all his bills. Every bill he had ever had in his life was wrapped up in elastic bands in shoe boxes, labelled *paid* and *unpaid*. I mean every receipt for every payment on every purchase was in there.

'The only food left in his fridge was a litre of milk and a jar of coffee.'

GRIEF

*What sort of mother, person, wife must I be for a child
of mine to kill himself? If I was good at all those things,
Collin would still be here ... Why why why why why?*

From the diary of Jan Schultz

Every death breaks hearts. But death by suicide is different.
The sadness of those left behind is almost unbearable because
it is so often intensified by guilt and shame.

The family feels exposed; there is the humiliation of being
somehow found wanting.

Julie Dunsmore, the New South Wales President of the
National Association for Loss and Grief, said that even when
families truly believed they had done all they could for their
child, they still had to deal with the looks, the innuendo and
the stigma which is associated with suicide.

Just as difficult to cope with is the common assumption
that people who kill themselves are at best unbalanced, at
worst, insane. There may be the suspicion of abuse, or the
inferred question: if this was such a loving, caring family,
why wasn't such unhappiness noticed?

'The trouble is that young people are fantastic at holding
up the mask that hides their true feelings,' said Julie
Dunsmore. 'There's a conspiracy of silence about the games
that are played to protect or deceive parents. A young person
may love their family very much and not want them to be

hurt. They miss the point when they decide that by killing themselves the family will be better off without them.

'They think "They'll get over it,",' which is an indication of his – or her – chronic lack of self-appreciation.'

If a suicidal young person has been very angry and their death was a way of getting back at the world, people don't want to talk about it. As a community we're not very good at dealing with anger, whether it's the anger of a young person out of control of his world or the anger of the parents who have lost their son or daughter.

There is no acceptable way for people to vent their anger in our society. When their rage is at its worst, some troubled boys become destructive and end up in the Juvenile Justice institutions. But most young people don't release their anger in a violent way at all. Instead they turn it inwards and upon themselves. It becomes depression.

'That's when we lose them,' said Julie Dunsmore, 'if not to suicide, to hopelessness and despair and all that comes from that.'

When their child commits suicide, parents are likely to feel totally rejected. Their son or daughter has betrayed them by choosing to die rather than staying in the life they gave them ...

And their arms are empty. The absence of their boy or girl becomes a physical pain. The child they have lost may have been in his early twenties, a big son who sometimes gave them a bear hug. They may not have had a hug for a long time because of the way he had changed, because of the trouble – but he was still their baby. They have lost the future – the fantasy that he was going to get his act together, to settle down, to give them grandchildren.

I cannot comprehend what it will be like when I am ten or fifteen years older and will not have seen him for

such a long time. I want to look at his photos, feels his
face, touch him ...

Diary of Jan Schultz

There is guilt too, in the fact that sometimes, when the anguish, the threats, the tantrums, the vandalism, perhaps even the arrests, have gone on for months or years, some parents may have a sense of relief. There is a limit to how much trouble even the most selfless parents can take before they crack. When the grieving sets in, it may be grief for the child they wanted who never, in reality, existed.

The railway track ran right past our backyard and sometimes, when he was quiet, he would go out and watch the trains. He had been mentally ill ever since he was a child, in and out of hospitals, having treatment which never worked because he was smoking marijuana which only made him worse, but he couldn't see it. He regularly threatened to kill himself. One day last year he told me that he was planning to throw himself under one of the trains. 'If you must do it, son,' I said, 'don't take others with you. Think of the driver, the passengers, how it would ruin their lives.' There was no point in pleading with him not to die. I knew that sooner or later, he would.

Lyn Williams*, whose son, Peter, hung himself in 1995,
aged twenty-five

GOOD GRIEF

There is nothing good about losing a child through suicide. But there are ways to handle grief.

The acknowledgment and release of anger is an important part of the grieving process. Many people find that before they can begin to cope with their great sadness, they need to release their rage.

They may find the need to rant and rave against God, against the community, against the health system, against themselves, against those closest to them, against their children's friends.

Often they are angry with the young person who has died. As heartbroken, as inconsolable, as torn apart as they are, they may find they are furious with their dead son or daughter. How could they do this to them? At this time? In this way? They gave this person life and he or she threw it away. And in such a way. How could they?

Yet how can they tell anyone they feel this way? They are expected to be sad, not angry. Nobody would understand.

Releasing the anger can bring some relief if it is done with care in a number of ways. An effective outlet for many parents, brothers and sisters, is writing letters to those with whom they are angry. These letters, however, must *not* be posted, because many regret what they have said or done at the height of their rage, hurting the people they love very much. Sometimes it is helpful to write a letter to the young person who died. What may begin as an emotional ordeal can release feelings and clarify issues which even now, still worry them.

Another way of letting out the anger is through physical release, like pounding pillows or belting phone books with a piece of solid rubber hose. The use of sound can be helpful. Going down to the surf and screaming at the waves, putting music on at full blast and shouting or singing at top volume provides a wonderful release of tension.

These are strategies which have been around since the invention of the wheel but for some people they work well.

Exercise is another effective outlet for the intense feelings of grief. Many people find simply getting out of the house and walking provides the different focus they need. Relaxation, crying, laughing and certain physical activity releases endorphins, which are the body's natural pain killers. People who are able to run, walk, swim or smash a ball around a court find it takes the edge off the pain, at least for a while.

At a support group bereaved people can say whatever they like without being judged, without some well-meaning loved one saying: 'Now, now, you know that's not how you really feel.' Of course it's not how they feel *all the time* but that's the other reason people won't release their anger. They are afraid of being misunderstood – that others will interpret their whole relationship with the young person who has died as being one of anger, and that they will say: 'Well, that's why he killed himself. Look how angry you are. Look how unapproachable you are. Imagine what it must have been like at home'.

THE EXPERIENCE OF GRIEF

I seem out of control of myself – my thoughts, my feelings, my actions. I feel frightened – I would love to go to hospital and to be just left alone, to have no one worrying about me and therefore be able to really let myself go down the slide to oblivion, into the big black hole of sadness …

Diary of Jan Schultz

Therapists talk about the four Fs of stress in crisis situations. These are:

- Flight – the need to run away, to get away from everything, especially other people, especially the pain; the desire to go off and start again and pretend none of this ever happened.

- Fight – the urge to hit out, to put your fist through a wall; men who have never done so go to the pub and start a fight; parents find themselves shaking their surviving children; people get into cars and drive like maniacs with no idea where they are going or why and no concern about safety or danger.
- Freezing – people feel numb and cold, unable to make decisions, unable to face the world. If this feeling goes on for too long it may damage not only relationships but the ability to study or work; it holds back the healing process.
- Fornication – Young people talk about 'stress bonking'. There is a need for release, to forget for a short time, to be held and cared for. Sexual activity may meet this need. Parents sometimes feel guilt because in having sexual intercourse they are likely to be enjoying themselves – and sex is linked with the conception and creation of life, which brings home the reality of the loss of their child.

How do people keep going?

'For a long while they are simply on automatic pilot,' said Julie Dunsmore. 'It's a matter of getting through each day.

'For those who have lost a child through suicide, learning to live with the loss is like learning to walk again. Although their wound is not visible, these men, women and children have to be treated as if they have had a really horrendous physical accident. So you don't expect those people to get on with their lives and pretend nothing has happened.'

If a person has agreed to counselling, they can talk about the way they feel to someone who is there purely to listen, to support, to encourage and to believe. But counselling sessions rarely run over an hour. Sooner or later they must leave their counsellor's office and face the world again.

'We ask them to set small goals for themselves,' said Julie Dunsmore. 'There's getting up, having a shower, what they will do that day, what they will say to people, how they will handle it if they become overwhelmed with their grief; what they are going to do when they see someone cross the street rather than speak to them, what they will answer if someone asks them how many children they have, what they will do if their other children come home from school upset at what people have been saying about their brother or sister.'

Julie Dunsmore encourages her patients to keep a daily diary in which they rate each day out of ten. This way they may see that each day fluctuates, that every day is not the worst.

'It's also a way for them to realise that this is not a process of getting over something and forgetting it. It's a new world. They will never be able to go back to the old one because for them, the death of this young person has changed everything. There are no magic wands to bring back the past.'

In trying to make sense of what has happened, some people blame themselves. They may look back into their history to find a reason why they should be punished in such a cruel way. They go over and over the 'what ifs' and 'if onlys', only to find reasons which make no sense to others. Nevertheless, their guilt and blame needs to be expressed because this is the only way their irrational beliefs can be challenged; only then can they work out what to do with the guilt that doesn't go away.

Many people feel so guilty that they expect to be punished. Their unhappiness can become their punishment. 'I ask them how long their sentence is going to be,' said Julie Dunsmore. 'When will their punishment stop? I challenge their belief that they must feel the pain all the time, that the intensity of their pain is equal to the love they felt for their child.'

Young people in mourning

There is no competition in grief. Heartache cannot be measured or weighed. The amount of pain that a person feels does not equal the amount of love they had for the one they have lost. For young people as well as the families of the bereaved, the loss of a friend through suicide is a wound that may never fully heal. It can have a huge influence on the way they see themselves.

'I see a lot of young people who have lost friends through suicide,' said Julie Dunsmore. 'Theirs is a disenfranchised form of grief. Many people have rules about who is entitled to grieve. It's as if a parent or a partner, or a brother or sister has a reason to grieve, but society puts a lesser value on the grief of friends.'

In fact when a young person suicides it has an incredible impact on their friends. They frequently feel betrayed, abandoned and helpless. Most need a chance to work through these feelings so they don't fester and complicate their way of dealing with their own lives.

'It really does affect their sense of who they are, and makes them question whether they're an okay person,' said Julie Dunsmore. 'They can become afraid of getting close to anyone else, for fear of being let down again. They too, can feel very angry. And frightened. They may think they understood how this person was feeling; perhaps they looked up to their friend as somebody who knew the answers. Yet his or her way of dealing with life, in the end, was to opt out. They ask themselves: "Am I going to do that too? Will it happen to me? Maybe I could have done something".'

Even if the person who died was not a really close friend, young people touched by suicide begin looking at those around them for signs of distress. They start reassessing their friends, especially those with problems, those who may be having relationship difficulties or troubles at home. They live with a sense of panic. The safety net of their world has fallen in, just at a time when they are trying to work out who they are in this world.

Their grief may be intensified if they are shut out and away from the family's sorrow and the funeral rituals. 'Families often close ranks after the death of a child,' said Julie Dunsmore, 'even more so with suicide, sometimes because of their shame, other times because of the preciousness of the funeral being the last contact with their child.'

SADNESS AND HEALING

Yet despite their pain and sorrow, families and friends survive. Time passes. Wounds slowly heal. Small shoots of hope spring from the branches of the family tree. Life goes on.

'Some people feel guilt even about healing,' said Julie Dunsmore. 'Finding a way to heal the pain of loss after the suicide of a young person is not easy. There are no quick fixes, or easy recipes to follow. The most difficult part of grieving is experiencing the pain, of feeling out of control. Support from caring people, a chance to have time to sit and experience their grief, the opportunity to revisit their memories of the young person who died – not just the tragedy but the other aspects of their life as well – has helped many through the pain of grief. To allow the tears to fall, to speak openly about their memories, to say the young person's name out loud, to be able to remember, to laugh about good times shared – all this helps people to come to terms with their new reality.

'While part of them may feel as if it has died along with the one they have lost, the healing is often about finding that part of themselves which can embrace life once again.'

MAZ: FEBRUARY 19

Maz spent her lunch break wandering around the air-conditioned shopping plaza where she worked, looking at baby clothes and dreaming of the future. First the land, then the house, then the baby. This time she would do everything in the right order. It would mean staying in the Unit of Destruction for a few more months maybe, but that might not be a bad thing right now. Her mother could do with a bit of moral support, while the old man was being such a bastard.

But at least she would have something to look forward to; she had a plan. She would be in control of her life. At last.

Danny rang her at the shop at 2 p.m. to tell her their application for a loan had been turned down. Their deposit wasn't big enough and they didn't have any security. Even combined, their wages were too low to make the repayments.

They were going to have to wait.

It was all right for Danny to say that, thought Maz as she put down the phone. He could wait with his posh plummy parents in their quiet carpeted house. She would have to sit out her time at the Fight Flat, the Home of Hate, the Unit of Destruction.

What did Danny know or care? He was just a kid, anyway. He probably wouldn't even know how to give her a baby. After all, he hardly ever touched her. Well, why would he want to? She was so fat and ugly. In fact they probably hadn't turned down the loan at all. He probably just said that, because he didn't really love her at all and didn't want to be stuck with her.

She had a horrible headache. Her limbs felt like lead. She was sick, that was the trouble. She probably needed to go to the doctor. She was sick in the stomach and sick in the heart. It was all she could do to drag herself off the stool and out the back where the other sales girl was sorting stock.

'I'm not feeling well,' said Maz. 'I have to go home. Can you manage on your own?' The girl was new. She looked startled. 'I don't know,' she said. Maz sighed and rang the owner of the shop. Luckily she was home. She said she'd be there as soon as she could.

While she was waiting, Maz took her mother's repeat prescription for sleeping tablets out of her wallet and handed it in at the pharmacy opposite.

Half an hour later she left the shop, collected the tablets and walked out of the centre. It was a hot, lazy February afternoon. Everybody seemed to be operating in slow motion. Maz walked to the station and bought a one-way ticket to Central Station. She was going away. No matter what happened, she was not going back to the hell that was home.

The train took a long time to come. The journey took longer. She looked out of the window at the long brown lines of ugly houses. The sky was filled with smog. The train rattled on the tracks. Not a nice place to be. Not a nice place. Not a nice place to be.

Why would you bring babies into this hole anyway? Why would you want to bring more kids into such a hopeless world which looked as if it was going down the toilet anyway? Why would you want to stay here at all?

What baby would want a person like you for a mother?

When she reached Central she went to buy a ticket to somewhere else. She couldn't think where. Her head was heavy. The decision was too hard. She left the station and walked through the tunnel. Everybody looked angry. The buskers were singing a miserable song. You couldn't blame them.

She found a pub and went in. She ordered a whisky and Coke and drank it quickly. It took longer to drink the second, but her head seemed to be clearing. It was dim and hot inside. She fumbled in her handbag for the pills. Glancing up, she saw the barmaid staring at her with blank, uncomprehending eyes. She reminded Maz of Bimbo Elizabeth. She sipped her drink and swallowed one tablet and then a couple more. It was no trouble. It was going to be easy.

They'd all be better off without her. This would just put an end to the worry. Next time the old man smacked her mother she wouldn't be there to hear it. She wouldn't have to race into the kitchen feeling helpless and sick, getting there too late to kill him because he'd gone straight out, slamming the door. With Maz out of the way Mum might finally throw him out and then she could live happily ever after with the saintly Jilly. They wouldn't want her around, causing more trouble for everyone. They wouldn't have to kill off any more of her babies or tell any more lies about her.

She knew they all thought she was just like her father.

They'd be better off without her and later on, everything would be sorted out.

There was nothing a few pills and a nice long sleep couldn't cure.

And there would be no mess.

Edward was in Sydney, doing work experience for his university degree. He was staying with a friend in the city, which was infinitely more pleasant than going home.

There was no phone in the office he was borrowing. He took the personal call at the reception desk in the outer office. 'Marilyn has been rushed to hospital in an ambulance,' said his mother. 'Apparently she has taken an overdose of something. I can't contact your father. Can you go and find out what this is all about?'

Edward swayed slightly as he hung up the phone. Involuntarily the elegant young receptionist put out a hand to steady him.

'Bad news?' she asked.

'I have to go,' said Edward. 'My sister has just tried to kill herself.'

The girl snatched back her arm. 'Oh my God,' she gasped. Edward flushed. Why had he said that? This wasn't something you talked about to people. His mother would kill him.

When Maz slumped into unconsciousness in the hotel booth, the barmaid had called an ambulance. Maz was taken to casualty and treated without delay. She was lucky, the doctor on duty told Edward. Suicide attempts usually took place late at night when resources were stretched. Maz had very sensibly tried to die in business hours.

She looked so small when he saw her and still so pretty, despite the ludicrous haircut and all the holes in her ears. They had taken away all the earrings and jewellery she wore like armour against the world. She looked young and vulnerable and pure, a baby with a flushed face, sleeping under a white sheet on a hospital bed. Maz, his little sister, nineteen years old and with a lot more living to do. Whether she wanted to or not.

She woke up several times during the night and he helped her stagger to the toilet, but she didn't recognise him. Around midnight their father arrived.

'You can go home,' Edward said. 'I'll stay. I don't mind it here.' His father hesitated. He was beautifully turned out in a lightweight double-breasted suit, a cream shirt and a silky tie in shades of mauve. One lock of hair had escaped from its moussed wave and hung over his forehead. Edward wondered if he had pulled it down on purpose.

'Is Mum coming?' asked Edward.

'No,' said his father. Did he actually have tears in his eyes as he gazed down at Maz on her austere white tray? 'She's staying home with Jilly. I don't want them upset any more than is necessary.'

Edward wanted to laugh at such pomposity. 'Gosh no,' he said, richly sarcastic. 'Whatever you do, you mustn't *upset* them.'

His father took his gaze away from his daughter and glared at his son. 'I used to be proud of you, you know,' he said. 'I used to be proud of all of you. That was all I wanted – kids I could be proud of.'

Edward stared back at his father for a long time while he gathered the courage to reply. 'That's funny,' he wanted to say. 'We were never proud of you.'

It would have been a great line. It would have made him feel a little better. But because this is a true story, and not a soap opera, he didn't say it. Edward always thought ahead. He was sickeningly aware of the repercussions which could flow from any words or behaviour that might anger his father. It was his mother who would pay, his mother, whom he loved deeply and admired more than anyone he'd ever known; his mother, fighting her exhausting battle for the respectability and contentment for which she had yearned all her life. And losing, always losing, although not because of the girl who lay here beside him. Not because of her.

So he said nothing.

This was the way it had always been with Edward.

His father left, tomato-nosed, without another word and Edward covered his face with his hands.

When he woke from a light doze, Maz was looking at him through her thick black lashes. 'So I stuffed that up too?' she said.

Edward grinned sadly and nodded.

Maz patted herself gingerly on the belly.

'They pumped my stomach?'

He nodded again.

'It's a fucking lousy way to diet,' she said, with a tremulous little smile.

Tears squirted from his eyes like fountains. She was so young and lovely, so vivacious, funny, cheeky and bold. She was everything he had never been and he couldn't bear to think that he had almost lost her.

Seeing him cry made her cry too. 'They took away my baby, Edward,' she sobbed.

'I didn't know,' he said. 'Mum only told me yesterday. That was a very bad thing they did to you.'

She stared at him as if she had never seen him before and he leaned over the bed and put his arms around her. 'I don't want you to die, Maz,' he choked. 'I love you, don't you know that?'

'Well actually,' said Maz, with her face against his tear damp neck, 'I suppose I do.'

Edward took her away for a holiday. She told him about the Unit of Destruction and he knew she couldn't face going back there for a while. They walked and talked for hours and ate a lot of delicious non-fattening food.

One night they ate with a group of young men who were staying in the same hotel and watching Maz dance with one of them afterwards, Edward was appalled at the way she clung to this virtual stranger, the uninhibited manner with which she coiled her arms around his neck.

How do you teach a girl to ration her loving, he wondered? Why did Maz always give so much so soon? When he mentioned it later she looked at him with something approaching pity. 'I'm not buttoned up like you, Edward,' she said. 'It's just me. I can't help it.'

When they returned, Edward rang the counselling service whose number was on a card the hospital had given him. Counselling was not easy to get and not only because of their mother's stony opposition. First they had to wait ages for an appointment. Then Maz decided she hated her first counsellor, who reminded her of a vampire. The second one fell pregnant after a few fairly productive weeks and Maz was unreasonably jealous. The third one, from a private clinic, smelled like her father and in any case, cost far too much.

Edward finally managed to get in touch with Diana James, who had been transferred to another high school but was able to recommend a colleague in practice at a government funded youth health centre. She thought Maz would like this woman and she's been right. Counsellor number four is working out well.

There was a bit of a setback when Maz found out Danny had been forbidden from seeing her any more. He told her his mother had warned him about being involved with anybody who was a mental case. She rang Edward and they talked about it. She rang Edward a lot. The phone bills to Melbourne cost more than a new wardrobe but their father didn't dare complain. Sooz remained a good friend and Jilly started to come out of her shell. From Maz's point of view, Jilly seemed to have grown up overnight, although she had an unsuspected chip on her shoulder about her sister always being the centre of attention. *Maz* the centre of attention? How ludicrous!

'Always,' said Jilly. 'Right from when we were tiny.'

'That shows you how wrong you are,' said Maz. 'Because I was *never* tiny.'

Maz started working part-time at a toy shop, which she really enjoyed. People always took to Maz. But at the back of her mind she was thinking seriously about going to university and studying nursing. Edward had suggested it. Good old Edward. All this time someone had cared about her after all.

CLUB SPERANZA: THE HOPE CLUB

Probably the most unique organisation to grow from the tragedy of suicide is Club Speranza.

The initials stand for Suicide Prevention Education Research Australia New Zealand Action; they make up the word *speranza* which in Latin languages means hope.

In an unusual initiative, Club Speranza is bringing together families who are bereaved by suicide and people who have attempted suicide. As Australia's first national consumer alliance, Club Speranza is uniting these people with professionals, service providers, researchers and welfare organisations, all of whom share the mutual goals of minimising suicide, providing support and comfort for bereaved friends and families and promoting good mental health.

The founders of Club Speranza, Tony Humphrey and Carol Jefferson, have both lost children to suicide.

'Suicide doesn't usually happen in business hours,' said Tony Humphrey, 'and neither does overpowering grief. We know that very often professional services are stretched, not available at the time or unable to respond in an appropriate way. Because of this, Club Speranza aims to provide personal support from people who, because of their own experience, understand this sort of situation. The club encourages survivors of the tragedy of suicide to offer each other support and understanding.'

Club Speranza operates on the premise that it is the people who have attempted suicide who are the real 'survivors' of the tragedy. It is essential, said Tony Humphrey, to convince these men and women that they are valued individuals and not cowards or traitors. At the same time, club members who have lost family members to suicide are fortified by the experience of helping others, while gaining a better insight into state of mind from which their loved ones may have been suffering.

Club Speranza advocates the introduction of **an easy three digit telephone number** for immediate access to professional health services and **friendship centres** where people who have attempted suicide and may have been receiving treatment for mental illness, as well those bereaved by suicide, can take time out to heal.

Club Speranza spreads its message through public meetings and referrals from health professionals. With groups now established in most states, its aim is to form a national chain of clubs whose representatives will work with government and non-government organisations, such as Lifeline, to give suicide survivors a chance to have their experiences and opinions heard.

QUESTIONS

Why did Collin Schultz and Jason Connor commit suicide?

Why did Maz try?

Why should we care?

They were not your own children, or mine. We never touched their skin, or stroked the hair from their foreheads, or squeezed their feet to check the growing room in their brand new shoes. We never wiped their eyes or heard their spelling or gripped them tightly to keep them safe from falling from lookouts, from tumbling off bikes, from drowning in deep water, from being squashed in crowds, from wandering onto busy roads, from all the dangers that once threatened to take them too early from life.

It's so easy, because they were not your children, or mine, to distance yourself at your desk, to read the facts, to consider the research, to draw logical conclusions. It's so simple to pick out a pattern, to work out an answer, to make a judgement on other people's lives.

Once we are personally touched by suicide, it's no longer easy. Once we see the shed it's impossible to escape the painful image of how Collin died there. Once we are faced with the reality of a boy taping up the windows of his car so that his lungs would fill with poison, once we are forced to imagine a young man actually sliding a noose over his head, pulling a trigger, facing a charging train, climbing a cliff and jumping into cold night space onto rocks many metres below … once we try to comprehend this degree of pain and desperation, it gets hard.

If we can see the evidence of the blade which sliced a girl's soft wrist; when we hear explanations from the same lips which consumed a murderous cocktail to escape from the agony of life, it gets a whole lot harder.

Once we meet the families and friends, once we hear about the fun and laughter in their lives as well as their worries, their problems and their deaths or attempts to die, we realise there are no answers, no judgements and no wise conclusions at all. We are left instead with too many questions.

Did Collin Schultz die because he felt inferior to his sisters and his friends? Because he couldn't read? Because his father was strict and uncompromising? Because he couldn't sort out his problems without his mother's help? Because despite his physical strength and dexterity, he despised physical violence? Or was afraid of it? Because he drank too much? Because he smoked pot? Because he didn't know how to extricate himself from a turbulent relationship? Because he believed the police were picking on him?

Did he die, as his broken hearted mother believes, because his family was too damned *nice*?

And Jason Connor? Did he kill himself because he could not come to terms with being Aboriginal? Because he wasn't Aboriginal enough? Because he had once been too fat? Because he was now too thin? Because he never recovered from the disappointment of finding out that Peter was not his real father? Because he missed his 'nanna', the one person who made him feel absolutely special? Because the thought of tracing his roots frightened him? Because he hated his job? Because he owed money? Because at twenty-four he felt burdened with responsibility for his sisters' happiness? Because he was lonely and had never had a girlfriend? Because he saw so much sadness in the people with whom his mother worked? Because his standards of cleanliness were so high that he could never be satisfied? Because life in that small mountain town held no promise for a boy like him? Because he never told anyone how unhappy he really was?

Did he die because he had been smoking marijuana regularly for years and a three week break from the drug had resulted in a chemically-induced depression which was no longer balanced by artificial 'highs'?

Did Maz empty a bottle of sleeping pills down her throat because her parents hated each other? Because her family had moved too many times for her to establish a secure peer group? Because she had been sexually promiscuous from a young age and felt worthless and unloved? Because she drank too much? Because she smoked marijuana? Because she thought she was adopted? Because she felt she couldn't live up to her mother's standards? Because she was ashamed of her father? Because the bank turned down her loan application? Because she was mourning for the baby which had been taken from her?

Or did Maz attempt to take her life in an effort to attract and hold the attention of a mother and a father who in her opinion, were too absorbed in their own difficulties, to notice hers?

The answer to all these questions is probably Yes.

And No.

Few if any suicides are the result of one single cause. All of the problems experienced by Collin, Jason and Maz have happened in some combination or another to other young people, who have overcome these and other even more horrific situations, and survived.

What these three young people had in common, not only with each other but with the vast majority of all young people who commit or attempt suicide, was their depression, a state of mind which developed during their childhood and adolescence and eventually resulted in their inability to cope with the present or to envisage any comprehensible future. Their condition, which was almost certainly exacerbated by their alcohol and marijuana use, had continued untreated and unresolved for months and probably years.

The other thing they had in common with each other and many other suicidal young people was that they couldn't talk to their parents about the way they were feeling.

Ruth Anderson, whose son, Adam, died in 1996, believes the disinclination for young people to talk to their parents results from their inability to come to terms with the inevitable breaking of the parent-child bond. 'They want to grow up and become independent of you,' she said, 'but as that starts to happen, they may find that it's harder than they thought. They long for some comfort and reassurance from you, but they are disappointed in themselves for needing that. So they take out their anger by distancing themselves from the family. They are in a sort of no-man's land between adolescence and adulthood and I now realise that even though they don't show it, they still have a desperate need to know how much you care about them.'

Collin, Jason, and Maz all had friends who were well aware of their desperate unhappiness; in the case of Maz and Collin, their friends knew they had made previous attempts on their lives. Nobody told.

However much Collin, Jason, Maz and Adam too, believed their parents loved them, they were convinced they would not understand.

Perhaps they were right.

'JUST HOW DO YOU COMMUNICATE WITH YOUNG PEOPLE?'

By listening to them.

Every book or article that has ever been written about living with adolescents and every professional who is willing to advise parents about their problems with kids, advocates good communication. Keep the communication lines open, we are told. Be around when they want to talk. Take advantage of every situation — the car, the dinner table, the end of their bed (as long as they are in it at the time) to encourage them to communicate with you.

Perhaps one of the reasons parents find it so hard to talk to their adolescents and grown children is that their idea of communicating is very different to that of the kids. Communication doesn't mean parents talking and young people listening and obeying. Successful communication may not involve much talking at all. What about the telephone, the most basic tool of communication in society today? We speak into it. But we achieve very little if we don't stop talking from time to time and listen as well – if only to ensure that the person at the other end of the line has heard and understood what we have said.

Good communication happens when the kids as well as the parents have a turn to speak, but also when kids as well as parents feel that what they say has been heard – *really* heard and considered.

As our children grow up it becomes increasingly important to hear what they are saying to us. Listening well is not easy in this busy world of ours. It takes time and patience. It may require several attempts to draw the young person out. It may even require an appointment – 'let's sit down together when we both get home tonight and you can tell me about the problem'. Or perhaps it's not a problem at all, just something that has come up. Good communication means sharing the good stuff as well as the bad. Talking things over with the oldies should never be something that only happens when there's a serious issue at stake.

Talking is terrific when it happens and even better if everyone gets an equal share of the lines. Listening, watching and caring play a big part in communicating as well.

It's as important to be aware of young people's behaviour, of the small signs, the changing habits, the body language, the attitudes to their friends, studies, music, interests, which give those closest to them an indication of how they are feeling about their lives.

Communication doesn't have to mean understanding, just as listening to young people doesn't mean we have to agree with them. It simply means we are interested in them and we respect the fact that they have views which are independent of ours. Few parents and their almost-adult children understand each other completely but why would they want to? The generation gap is as essential to society as hot runny butter is to toast. It makes life juicy and interesting. How boring the world would be if our kids thought just like us.

Simply caring enough to listen and sympathise, without jumping in to advise or judge, would be a big step forward in many families.

In an ideal world, young people would confide serious trouble to their parents. But even in a close family, this doesn't always happen. Adolescence is a time for re-evaluating relationships and testing autonomy. Despite having a warm and loving relationship with their families, young people may want to break away, to establish themselves as independent individuals. They may not *want* to tell their mother or father when they feel upset or unhappy.

Parents alone cannot be lumbered with their children's state of unhappiness, whatever may have caused it. The emotional health of their child may well be out of parents' hands. Their son or daughter might require the sort of professional care that they are not qualified to give. Parents need help when it comes to recognising that the situation is serious enough for specialised treatment and a doctor's assessment.

This is why the role of qualified professionals is a vital one when dealing with seriously depressed young people. It's why all of us must share the responsibility for finding the solutions.

ANSWERS

Too many young Australians are leaving life early. We've looked at which ones are the most likely to commit suicide and we've examined the reasons why. So now what? The answers lie in finding those who need help before many more of our young people die; in being prepared to throw ourselves into the growing heap of their shattered hopes and putting together something that resembles a decent future for them; in providing them with the spirit and the strength all men and women need to overcome the disappointments and disillusions that are a part of life.

How do we do this? Does anybody know? Who is willing and able to provide some answers to the questions youth suicide leaves behind?

THE MENTAL HEALTH DIRECTOR: PROFESSOR BEVERLEY RAPHAEL

Professor Raphael is the Director of the Centre for Mental Health in the New South Wales Department of Health.

'There are things we can change and there are things we can't. But I believe there is a lot we can do.

'We should ask the young people themselves a lot more questions and listen to their answers. As professionals we are often afraid to hear their words. Yet how can we develop programs to help them if we don't learn from their experience rather than ours?

'Government health departments should be aiming at establishing help for young people and their families at a local and community level; to let them know who to call when they have a problem; to enable them to benefit from someone else's experience.

'We have to strengthen community responsiveness to young people who need help. But not only that. Families have to be involved too.

'First of all you have to take on broader social issues like youth unemployment. Without employment they have no sense of opportunity, no chance to test themselves out as independent adults in a community situation. Even if their families can support them or if they can get the dole, it doesn't give them any sense of personal value.

'But work isn't everything. If they can't work, what other things are there which can add value to their lives?

'We have to look at preventive programs aimed at promoting resilience in young people so that they don't have to keep on suffering and proving themselves over and over again.

'They have to have rewarding experiences at school and at home. They have to be encouraged actively to be involved in those different experiences and given a sense of achievement instead of having their efforts devalued.

'We have to put positive parenting programs in pre-schools. The resources for young people's programs are too often withdrawn because results may not be immediate; there is not enough recognition that our children are the future.

'There is a lot parents can do. Young people's problems are serious. They are not spoilt and manipulative; it's not a joke. They need help. To provide that adults have to set aside their own needs and listen. A lot of people are no longer prepared to do that, but that's what having children is about.

'As parents, we have to look at what we value as achievements – not just medals for excellence in a particular field or sport, but a broader spectrum of achievements in many different ways.

'We have to look for the worth in our young people. You don't have to get it by sending them to private schools or spending heaps of money on them. You can do so much yourselves, at home. It's a matter of stopping and thinking – not flying off the handle. It's a matter of parents asking themselves *why* their young person is being difficult.

'They have trouble with their relationships because they are young and inexperienced. Sometimes you have to accept their hate and rage and let them get it out and stay with them, listening, not judging them. That's what therapists charge people money to do. Parents can do it for nothing. It's their job. The rewards for that sort of patience are in the future.

'Previous generations looked forward to job security and the permanence of marriage, children, grandchildren. It's a changed world now and the older generation has to be careful not to saddle young people with their expectations – or their current disappointments. Their world cannot be the same as ours. The future they will inherit is not likely to be the same as it was for us.

'People are no longer going into a job after leaving school and staying with that company or even in that profession, for life. With at least one-third of couples getting divorced, changes in family structure are inevitable. Some blended families work; some don't.

'Adults tend to be very cynical about all of this. Instead of giving out pessimistic messages, we should be helping our young people cope with the inevitable changes that will occur in their lives. We have to give them something to replace the security that is no longer there.

'Mental health has its roots in childhood and adolescence. There are high levels of depression in young people. But kids get a second chance in their teenage years. That chance can be increased with positive prevention programs. They need emotional competence. They need to learn optimism. We should help them develop a fighting spirit, the feeling that they can manage, an empathy with others. It's very important to remember that good mental health is not about happiness; it is about coping well.

'We have to give them hope. After all, if people had always given in to grief and despair the human race would have died out long ago.'

THE CHILD PSYCHIATRIST: DR TITIA SPRAGUE

A child and adolescent psychiatrist at the New Children's Hospital in Sydney, Dr Sprague believes society must focus not only on intervention but on prevention.

'We need to catch these kids before they throw themselves off the cliff and into the sea. We will always have to station someone at the bottom, in the hope of catching them. But what we really need are a lot more people at the top, and indeed, miles from the cliff, finding the kids long before they even set their eyes in that direction.

'We have to start when the children are in primary school, or even pre-school. We protect them against infectious diseases at a very young age; we can also reach young children with programs which can protect them against depressive symptoms, despair and mental illness. We should be teaching them problem-solving skills, how to cope with relationships, how to evaluate the kind of faulty thinking patterns which people get into when they are depressed. We can stop them thinking things like: "Oh, this is never going to be any good", "I'm always going to be hopeless", "I'm hopeless at this so I'll be hopeless at everything else".

'It has to start when they are young because by the time they get to high school, some of the kids most at risk have detached themselves from getting anything from school anyway. Disruptive behaviour can be an early sign of depression and the best prevention programs for disruptiveness begin in pre-school. If there has been no intervention, by the time they are eight they are used to mucking up and the parents are used to yelling at them for mucking up; the pattern is set.

'Parents and teachers need to encourage children to take responsibility for their actions; they should recognise that everything they do has consequences. This is a juggling act because it is also important that children don't start thinking that if anything goes wrong, it must be their fault.

'A problem-solving program introduced to primary school children in Pennsylvania, in the United States resulted in a lower rate of depression among these children when they reached early adolescence. The program was devised by psychologists but conducted by classroom teachers. This is really exciting because it shows these ideas can work. Yes, it's more work for teachers but it comes down to priorities – as a society, we have to decide what are the most important things we should be teaching our kids. If it comes out that these are life-saving measures, surely their priority is worth bumping up a bit?

'It would be great if health professionals were able to work in with schools, by collaborating more with teachers and counsellors – especially in primary schools.

'Parents too, can teach kids about problem-solving, particularly when it comes to dealing with setbacks and relationship issues. If parents, when faced with a problem, declare that their whole life is a disaster or blame themselves for every bad thing that happens, then their children are likely to think that way too.'

THE BRAIN MAN: PSYCHOPHYSIOLOGIST, JOHN ANDERSON

John Anderson has been studying the effects of drugs and alcohol on the attitudes and intellects of young people.

'Programs preaching abstinence from alcohol and cigarettes are already operating in primary schools and even pre-schools. The children take no notice of them because they see adults, often their own parents, drinking and smoking. The message is confused or lost. If marijuana is deregulated we will have to forgive the kids for assuming this is a harmless drug as well.

'Children need to be educated from a very early age not to take drugs at all. They should be informed of the damage that alcohol, nicotine, marijuana and the other illegal drugs do to their bodies, both in the short and long term. We have to give them accurate information and graphic pictures of what is happening to their brains. This need not be done in an emotive way. They simply need to be provided with the facts.

'So-called harm minimisation won't work for the current generation of young people. It's too late.'

THE GRIEF COUNSELLOR: JULIE DUNSMORE

The New South Wales President of the National Association for Loss and Grief and a psychologist at Sydney's Royal North Shore Hospital, Julie Dunsmore has counselled many young people who have lost friends through suicide.

'There is an urgent need to teach young people how to help friends in distress. Adolescents are more likely to tell a friend about their deeper feelings. We need to teach young people how to deal with a friend's disclosure, because it is such a heavy responsibility for them.

'Their concern of course, is that by telling what they have heard, they will be betraying their friend – and dobbing is so frowned upon in Australian culture.

'We want young people to recognise despair and distress as something that is not right. We need to convince them that talking to an older person about what they know is a way of being a true friend. They can't be expected to make things right on their own.

'They need the right words when they are asked to keep a secret. Can you imagine a nineteen-year-old saying to his mate: "I care too much about you to keep this to myself?" A more likely response would be: "Don't be a stupid bastard" – or total silence.

'*We have to persuade them to tell. To tell and tell and tell until somebody listens.*

'While ninety percent of the young people who kill themselves are believed to have some degree of mental illness, very few of them are in therapy. This is despite the fact that depression, alcohol and drug dependence, schizophrenia and personality disorders are strongly associated with suicide. Even if they do seek help, health workers are too stretched to listen for long.

'The truth is that this has not been seen as a problem until quite recently. If someone has a clearly defined mental illness there is help available. But if a young person is troubled and hurting, but doesn't fit into any nice little category, then there are fewer professionals out there who can help them in a crisis, who have the time to talk to them and support them.

'Even if a health professional makes an appointment to talk to a young person in trouble, you can't do everything you need to do in an hour. Most GPs don't even have an hour – they would be hard pressed to give a young person twenty minutes.

'Some telephone help lines are effective, but there are many young people who would never in a pink fit ring a help line.

The majority of troubled students won't approach a school counsellor either. Boys don't as a rule go to counsellors. Men in general don't go to therapists. In another era it was acceptable for men to talk to priests or ministers – at least they were blokes and were prepared to listen to them. Counsellors have in many instances replaced confessors – but how do you get the young people to visit them?

'There must be a way of setting up a service totally independent of the school so that students can ask for help without having everyone in the school know about it. I believe we could do something with all these sports medicine clinics which are being established. Their services could be expanded to provide counselling, contraceptive advice and other services required by young people.

'The kids might go to a place like that, because it would not have the dreaded "mental health" label attached to it.

'We should be talking to young people who have attempted suicide. Parents' groups need to understand the way young people feel. Health professionals need to hear what the kids are saying about access to help and health facilities.

'There is a critical need in all states for wise, caring, educated adults who will listen, as well as trained teams of health workers who know what to do both in a crisis and in the long term.

'After all, suicide is the tip of the iceberg. So many lives are ruined by distress. The amount of kids who drop out of school, who end up in gaol, who actually become perpetrators of crimes because of this distress is a huge and expensive problem.

'Everybody is trying to blame everybody else. But I truly believe there is a need for everyone in the community – parents, teachers, health workers and the kids themselves – to support each other in this fight against young people's despair.'

THE YOUTH WORKER:
BARRY JOHNSON

The manager of Devonport Youth Accommodation Services in Tasmania, Barry Johnson, has been working with young people for twenty-six years.

'Kids talk to kids. We should be telling young people how to recognise when their friends are in trouble and how to respond effectively.

'Young people do care about each other. If they are shown what to do and told what to say, they can do a lot more good than any of us.

'Right now, if a kid tells his mate he is thinking of taking his life, the mate has no idea what to do. He or she feels uncertain – they don't know if their friend is bullshitting or if he is serious. But if that friend dies, they feel horribly guilty. They blame themselves for not acting, for not doing something about it.

'If they know what to do, what to say and who the appropriate adult is to tell, they will be prepared. If the friend still takes his life, at least they will know they've done everything they could to stop him.

'Suicide prevention should be incorporated into each school's individual living skills programs – that way the troubled kids will find out how to get help. We have to remember that these young people don't really want to die. They certainly don't want their friends to die. But they know it's happening.

'People say they don't want kids talking about it. But once it happens, you won't stop them talking about it. It would be much better if they talked about it before it happened so that they were aware of what they could do to stop it.

'If you cloak suicide in mystery it only makes it worse for the ones who are left behind.'

THE GOVERNMENT

The tragedy of youth suicide has been recognised by the Commonwealth and State governments.

Not before time. As Sydney psychiatrist, Dr Jean Lennane concluded in *The Australian* newspaper in January, 1997: 'Belatedly noticing a cull of our children is surely not the best way to find out there are problems with social and health policies.'

In July, 1995 the Commonwealth Department of Human Services and Health put into operation the 'Here for Life' youth suicide prevention initiative with funding of thirteen million dollars to be spent over four years. A Youth Suicide Prevention Advisory Group travelled to all states and spoke to many organisations in order to provide independent advice to the government on priorities and effective prevention schemes. With the change of government in March 1995, an election promise resulted in a new initiative, 'Giving Hope to Our Youth', and an additional eighteen million dollars to be distributed to selected programs over three years.

The state governments are financing their own programs. Each state has agreed to cooperate with the Commonwealth government in a networking initiative which will see the publication of a document which lists what projects are in operation, *what is working and what is not*. The professionals themselves sometimes admit that they are very slow to give up what feels right to them but is not working for the people. Both non-government and government organisations will be involved.

Competition for the government dollar is intense and in some circles, almost bitter. The way in which the Coalition Government has allocated the most recent funding has already been criticised by those youth suicide prevention educators who believe money would be better spent on long term prevention and awareness programs, rather than crisis intervention work. According to Barry Taylor, a member of the original Federal Government advisory group, since the government funding was announced, suicide prevention groups which once worked together have now stopped talking to each other. Everyone wants to have a go at reducing the youth suicide rate but nobody wants to share ideas or take it in turns.

What the professionals need to remember is that none of their prevention strategies will work if the kids won't play.

THE INTERNET

Reach Out! is the world's first fully interactive youth suicide prevention service available on the Internet. Because the 'net offers unparalleled opportunities to reach young people in need, the potential effectiveness of the service has been recognised and funded by corporate sponsors and by the Federal Government. It has been endorsed by suicide prevention specialists from Australia and overseas. Specifically tailored to three distinct audiences – young people, family and friends and professionals – Reach Out! provides a wide variety of services, including advice on warning signs leading to suicide, forums for sharing stories for young people who feel isolated and a detailed geographical guide to prevention services.

It is believed that forty percent of Australians aged eighteen to twenty-four have access to the Internet, which makes it an ideal tool to encourage interactive communication between young people in trouble and those who can help them. Reach Out! will be carefully screened to ensure it does not become a forum for suicide notes and methods of suiciding. The service, which has been established and designed by the New Australia Foundation, may well extend internationally. (See *Where to get help*, page 291.)

THE KIDS

Kelli, eighteen, was selected as the the 1997 Young Australian of the Year for Tasmania. During 1996 Kelli conducted her own research into youth suicide, approaching thirty schools, of which thirteen responded. (Several schools where a student had suicided turned her down.) She interviewed 4,000 students from Year Seven to Year Twelve. She has deferred her university studies for a year and is employed at a fast-food outlet which is making it possible for her to save some money while continuing her suicide prevention work.

'What kids need most,' said Kelli, 'is more information. If you explain what is going on and why and you tell them what to do, they will cope much better.

'It's rubbish to say that if you talk to kids about suicide it will put the idea into their heads. Kids talk about suicide a lot more than most adults would ever dare.

'Three percent of kids in trouble talk to teachers. Ten percent talk to their parents. Eighty percent talk to their friends. Unless you know what to do when a depressed friend talks to you about how they feel, they can drag you down with them.

'There must be adults kids can turn to if they or their friends are in trouble. They are perfectly aware that they can't help their friends. But they need to know what the warning signs are, how to react and who to go to for help.

'Right now young people don't talk to most adults. They are particularly loathe to talk to teachers as no matter what you say, teachers are right up there on some sort of pedestal and kids are ants on the ground. Most troubled kids believe if they talk to teachers it will be repeated in the staffroom and they will be regarded as being "different" which kids hate.

'If a young person is taken to a shrink and told they are mentally ill things get worse for them. The word "mental" makes them think they are crazy. All they need is lots of help. But then other parents say: "Take a couple of Panadol and have an early night". That's the other extreme.

'Young people today seem to attach too much importance to having a relationship with someone. Kids seem to feel unloved these days. I don't know whether it's because so many of them have parents who are both at work or parents who have broken up. I can't comment on that, really, as I am in a very happy family, even though there's just me and my mum and she has always gone to work. But so many kids feel they *must have* a boyfriend or a girlfriend. When that breaks up they don't know how to go on.

'Family breakdown plays a huge part in kids' problems today. So do drugs. Young people are supposed to have it easy in lots of ways but they have to be so much older and more responsible now than they used to be. Jobs have a lot to do with it too. You get told if you don't do well at school, if you don't get a university degree or if you're not *very* good at something, you'll be a nobody. Schools create enormous pressure.'

Jonathan, *sixteen, is the youngest in a Melbourne family of six children and is the only one still at school. He has had very little to do with youth suicide although like most boys his age, he has heard through friends of various young people who have taken their own lives.*

'I don't really agree with some of the solutions that have been suggested by the professional people. I don't know about having more counsellors – a lot of us don't feel comfortable with those sort of people.

'Some girls will talk to the school counsellors. I think it's very difficult to talk about serious stuff to people you don't even know.

'It's true that a lot of it comes down to having parents who talk to you and listen to you. That helps. But there are a lot of things you wouldn't want to discuss with your parents. If you had a really serious problem you'd be more likely to talk about it to your friends.

'Boredom is what's wrong with a lot of kids today. Sitting at home thinking too much won't make your problems go away. I can imagine it must feel pretty bad if you're never rewarded, if you feel you're not good at anything and you feel really bad about yourself. But if you get involved in sport or something you're good at, you feel much better. Sport – football in my case – gives you something to do with your time and when you play, you let a lot out. You stop worrying about what other people are thinking of you and you stop stressing. The best thing about sport is that you don't have to think about anything at all. You just play the game. Maybe there should be more activities for young people and more places for them to go where they can mix and have a good time together.

'I'm looking forward to the future. I've seen what my brothers and my sister have gone through to get jobs and I know it won't be easy. But the freedom will be great.'

Jaclyn, *nineteen, lost six friends to suicide in the two years from 1994 to 1996. Three of them were close friends. Jaclyn has spoken on the subject of youth suicide to scores of young people at conferences and seminars in Sydney. A student at the Australian Catholic University, she has also choreographed and performed a dance dedicated to the memory of her friends.*

'It may be cool for kids not to talk to their parents but a lot of parents don't want to talk to their kids. Life is so rushed and few adults take the time to find out what their children are doing after school, where they really are, who they are with, what they are thinking. They don't look at their school books or ask questions about what is going on at school or work or university. They don't get to know their kids' friends. These days most parents are both at work all week and at weekends they are out with friends or having dinner somewhere while the kids are left in charge of their own lives. In wealthy families the kids are given huge allowances but the parents have no idea how they spend their time and money. In working class families a lot of kids have the additional responsibility of preparing meals and looking after younger brothers and sisters because their parents are not there much.

'Some teachers speak to students in a way which utterly destroys their self-esteem. A lot of us don't trust the school counsellors, although we might talk to a friendly teacher.

'The result is that young people have a lot of worries, from fighting with their family and friends, to study, to money problems, to managing homework as well as their jobs. They don't like the way they look or feel. They just feel bad about themselves all the time and they think they can't live up to the standards their families and schools expect. They don't know who to turn to or where to get help. Their worries build up into a snowball which starts to roll, getting bigger and bigger and faster and faster as it goes down. They don't know how to stop it.

'My girlfriend hung herself in her garage. The boy who helped me choreograph my dance for my HSC assignment put rocks in his pockets and walked into the sea and drowned. None of the rest of us knew what to do. We were so angry and sad but we felt betrayed by the adults in our lives. Nobody had ever told us this could happen. Nobody told us what we could do for friends who were feeling this bad. Nobody told us where we could go to get help – or if there was any help available.

'The school counsellor told us to put it behind us and get with our own lives. We couldn't. It ate away at us. We wanted to talk about it together but they didn't encourage that. We wanted to read about it but there are no books on youth suicide in any school libraries.

'We desperately need more education on suicide prevention. There has to be people for us to talk to – but young people. Kids think anyone over twenty five is old and boring and they won't listen to them. Parents need to know more about it too.

'The help has to be there when you need it. There's an area youth service in an office near me. Every time I've passed it, it's been closed.

'I wish young people realised that the future is for them; that nobody knows what may be out there but we all have the power to make things happen for ourselves. No problem is so bad that it can't be fixed by talking to someone you trust. There are always solutions, even if you can't see them straight away.'

Solutions

- A greater commitment by PARENTS to their children, especially in giving them the time, care and attention they need, and in reducing marital conflict.
- More attention in SCHOOLS to encouraging young people to believe that the future is theirs to shape, and giving them faith in themselves to tackle this task.
- A more conscious effort by the MEDIA not to promote a culture of demoralisation and disillusion. The media MUST play a more positive and constructive role in young people's lives.
- Major POLITICAL reforms to make the processes of government more flexible and responsive to community needs. This includes moving beyond the contemporary political pre-occupation with economic growth and efficiency.
- A renewed SPIRITUALITY, a sense of being connected to the world and the universe in which we live that transcends individual needs and material things.

Compiled by: Richard Eckersley, Canberra, ACT, 1996

AFTER COLLIN

They went ahead with the wedding. 'I knew I would be grieving for my brother for a long time,' said Cathy. 'Whenever we had the wedding, Collin was still not going to be there.'

So three days after the funeral Cathy and Dean were married. The wedding photos are stiffly posed. The colours are bright but the faces are blank, like those in old-fashioned sepia photographs.

Eighteen months later, in answer to a terrible need, Jan went to the Gosford Court House and took out the file of Collin's death. There were some photographs there which she badly needed to see.

Jan wrote in her diary: 'The last photo was a shock at first. I couldn't look at it at first and I started to cry because it was a close-up of Collin's face. I had to make myself look first at only part of the picture with another photo blocking out his eyes. I gradually looked at the whole picture and was eventually able to study all the photographs. How I wanted to lift him out of those photos and hold him close. I just wanted to feel his skin, his hair.. I kept running my fingers over his skin and face, imagining what he used to feel like. It was my way of saying goodbye ... '

Jan's initial reaction to her son's suicide, however, was anger.

'I was very angry with Collin, with Ron, with the world in general. I was utterly pissed off with God. Being a Christian made it harder for me because one of my biggest worries was where Collin was. I'm sure other people would think that sounds weird but it wasn't weird to me. I don't know what happened in the last hours of Collin's life. Maybe he asked God to help him, I just don't know.

'It took me about three years to decide that Collin would be waiting there for me when I went to Heaven.

'I arranged for Julianne to have counselling almost straight away. I took her to a private clinic. It cost me one hundred dollars an hour and she went for about twelve months, but if I had to I would have sold everything we owned to get her that help. She was my main concern at the time; she started drinking and doing dangerous things with the car. Robbie was very worried about her behaviour. After a year she stopped going to counselling and never went back. She said the counsellor complained to her about another client and she figured that when she left he would probably do the same thing about her.

'I tried to go back to work. Some days I wouldn't get there but usually I was okay at the office. I would come home and fall apart. I didn't cook for two years. Ron took over all the meals. I cleaned. I became a manic cleaner. I've always enjoyed housework so that's what I did. Sometimes at 3 a.m. Three weeks after Collin died I covered a lounge. I had to keep doing things.

'I went to a suicide survivors self-help group. It helped to find out I wasn't alone.

'After about six months our world pretty much fell apart. I wanted to move out. I didn't want to be responsible for any other human being ever again. I didn't want to be the mother any more. I knew I had a good husband and three children but that wasn't what I wanted. I wanted Collin.

'I didn't want people depending on me. I kept wishing I had breast cancer so that I could die but nobody could blame me. I wanted to be put into hospital so that someone would look after me. At home, everything revolved around me. Ron kept asking me what I wanted. What I really wanted was to be away from him and everyone else. I thought I might get a little flat somewhere and the others could come and visit me now and then but I wouldn't be responsible for them all the time.

'I was very very angry with Ron. I kept thinking: "I hate Ron. I hate Ron. I hate Ron." I hashed over things he had said in the past, I blamed him for those times when I had allowed his opinion to override mine about things we did about Collin's problems.

'A friend recommended a counsellor at the district hospital. This didn't cost me anything and I think more people should know these services exist because without it, I would not have been able to survive. I counted the days to each visit. It was my lifeline.

'We have such good friends. We were never without somebody ringing us and checking to see how we were. I think they must have had a roster going. Not just women – men were doing it for Ron, too, which is unusual, I think. We are perhaps in the minority in that we didn't lose any friends when Collin died.

'But no matter how good your friends are, you can't keep saying the same things to them, over and over again. You can't keep endlessly talking about your dead son and your own feelings. It's not fair to them.

'You can say anything you like to a counsellor. I talked and talked and I cried a great deal. It's safe and it's neutral. A counsellor doesn't judge you when you say you hate God, you hate your husband, you hate yourself.

'I thought Ron was so cold, so hard. People would ask us how we were doing and he would always say: "We're going well now". I was so sick of this lie. I wanted to say: "We're hurting. We're struggling. There is this big black hole behind me and if I go back just one step, I might fall in and never get out again".

'After a long time Ron agreed to go to counselling too. He only went for a couple of months. I thought he needed help, though he would never admit it. But I also thought if he didn't soon start saying the right things to me then our marriage was in dire trouble.

'I went to counselling regularly for nearly three years. I talked out my anger. I was so angry with Collin. I had given him so much love, I had spent so much more time on him than I had on the others. I had worked so hard to get him the extra things he seemed to need. He had betrayed me.

'I was angry with him because of what his suicide had done to Ron and Julianne and Adam and Cathy. I was angry because he was never going to have children and I had always thought he would be the most marvellous dad. I was even furious about all the work and time we had put into his beautiful teeth!

'In the last few months I haven't felt like getting away from life unless things go wrong. As soon as that happens I feel desperate to get out. Of course I never go.'

For the first two years, Ron put all his energy into coping efficiently with a tragedy which was too horrific to cope with in any way at all.

'I was taken to church as a child but I fell out with it. It seemed to be that people only went when they were down and I decided that was hypocritical. That's why I didn't go rushing off to church when Collin died. But Jan's been going to a new church for the last couple of years and I've started going with her. I like it because nobody tries to brain wash me and a lot of things you've never understood get explained.

'For two years after Collin died I was ducking for cover while Jan lashed out. Her counsellors told her to say how she felt – and she did! The biggest arguments came out of the smallest things.

'My way of coping was to turn my head into the wind and to go forward. I never let myself look back. I thought only of the good times. I thought that was the right thing to do.

'I knew about Jan's black hole, but I had hold of her. I was there to pull her out if she needed me to. In the meantime I looked after my family as well as I could.

'After eighteen months she told me that if I wanted to save our marriage I had to go to counselling with her. That's why I went. If your marriage is threatened, you do anything you can.'

Cathy's marriage lasted two years. During that time her first love, Trevor, a pilot, was killed in a plane crash in South Australia. It was another blow for the reeling family who had loved this young man like a son.

When she decided to divorce her husband Cathy was pregnant. Her daughter, Saranna, was born in 1995 after suffering from a stroke while still within her mother's womb. She suffered damage to the right side of her brain. For nine months the baby was in constant pain; Cathy and her family, unable to relieve Saranna's agony, found themselves wrestling with a different sort of torture. Cathy, Jan and Ron devoted themselves to the baby and by her first birthday, with a change of medication and the intensive care and attention of her family, her future began to look brighter than it had when she first arrived in the world.

Cathy and Saranna now live back at home and Cathy works part-time as a scientific officer. She fought against counselling for several years, preferring to keep her pain inside; she finally decided to talk to a counsellor at the hospital where she worked and she believes this has helped. She is still inclined to think it's a pretty shitty world, but when Saranna's medication is keeping her well and when she sees her baby's fat, pink smile, and when she looks at her child in the arms of her doting grandfather, Cathy Schultz sometimes indulges herself in a little bit of hope.

Julianne didn't go back to school the year Collin died. On her first day of Year Twelve, the following February, she refused to read the text which had been set for the Higher School Certificate examinations. It was *The Crucible*; the cover featured a hangman's noose.

'I was angry with Collin for a long time. I reacted in a similar way to Mum. I found out a lot about his life that I hadn't known before, especially his learning difficulties.

'I think he was drunk and he had taken ... whatever he had taken ... and it was just a stupid thing he did.

'The reason I went into teaching is because kids need a better start in life than Collin had. Literacy is such an important issue and it is very closely linked with self-esteem. Children need to be taught to read and write properly when they are young but this has to be followed through. Teachers need to be aware of the effects that their teaching, in all its forms, can have on any student, regardless of age.

'My husband Robbie has dyslexia and they didn't pick that up either. He did an adult reading course which has made him feel much better. Collin would never have done that.

'When somebody commits suicide you have so many dreams where they are with you and everyone is happy and it was just one big stupid mistake they made. It's always so real and you wake up thinking they are back and they're not. You get so angry with them.'

'Our biggest concern now is Adam,' said Jan. 'I think anyone who has lost a child through suicide has this fear that their other children are also at risk. Adam is tall and handsome and although his hair is fairer, he looks more like Collin every day. For a while we were worried that he seemed to be modelling himself on Collin in almost every way. However, after we had all had some counselling, Ron and I became less paranoid; Adam has sold his hotted-up car and has bought an old, less obvious, one and he is trying to understand our feelings and fears for him.

'I have tried to change since Collin died. I try to be louder, to laugh more. I try to bake more. I used to always be shoving fruit down our kids' throats but it's cakes and treats they like. I have tried to lower our standards, to accept lesser values. But I can't. None of it has worked. I found out you can't change your personality. I was able to re-evaluate what I was doing but I think I got into even more trouble trying to change myself.

'What we *have* changed is the way we treat our children. These days we question ourselves constantly. We have no faith any more in our ability to make decisions for our kids. We did our best thing and it wasn't good enough.'

Sharon said she was dumbfounded by what Collin did. 'There had to be something wrong, didn't there? Why didn't he have any hope? I have hope. I have hope all the time.

'After he died I was a mess. My parents took me to England for six weeks. They were brilliant.

'Four months later I went into a local pub with my brother. Somebody said: 'God, look at that. Didn't take her long, did it?'

'At first I saw a lot of Collin's family but after a while I stayed away. I knew every time they looked at me they were reminded of him.'

Eighteen months after Collin's death, Sharon met John, with whom she now lives. He is the father of her children. 'I look at what other people do to their lives and I think: "I just want to have a happy family. I just want to be happy".'

Until the funeral was over, Jaakko felt as if a huge load was pushing him into the ground. His strict Pentecostal Church upbringing left him unable to cope with the thought of where Collin might be.

At the service he heard about Judas, the disciple who had hung himself after betraying Jesus. Judas, he learned, had been forgiven by God. 'It made me feel a bit better,' he said, 'knowing that Collin had probably been forgiven too.'

Jaakko himself, however, found it impossible to forgive the man who had bullied Collin on the last night of his life. He confronted him in a quivering rage, reducing him to tears of remorse. 'It was a long time before Lindy managed to convince me that what Collin had done he had done to himself.'

It took years, Lindy said, for Jaakko to get over the death of his friend. The rows, tears and heartache went on and on. Sometimes she thought his heart would never mend.

For twelve months there wasn't a day when he didn't think about Collin.

'What I worked out is that young people our age, they get themselves into a hole and they don't think they can get out again,' said Jaakko. 'They don't give it enough time. The thing is, bad things happen to most people but then you heal and you kick on. Kids today don't seem to realise there are bigger and better things out there.'

Jaakko and Lindy were married in 1995 after a seven-year engagement. Their first child, Rhianna, was born a year later.

'For us, these days,' Jaakko admitted, 'things are getting better all the time.'

Collin Schultz's HR Holden is now in the Holden Museum at Echuca, Victoria, a testimony to one young man's superlative skill, which has drawn the attention of qualified engineers and experienced mechanics from all over Australia.

LESSONS

'We have so many friends who thought we were "a lovely family",' said Jan Schultz. 'They try to tell me now that given that time again I would have changed nothing. That's not true. I would have done thousands of things differently and Ron would too. I don't think anyone who has lost a child through suicide could say they wouldn't change anything.

'Collin's life has been put under a microscope since he died. So has our parenting. And there is so much we would do differently.

'We would teach him how to stand up to us so that when he went out into the world he could stand up for himself. That doesn't mean fighting; it means believing in yourself. I think Collin thought he had to fight to get anything he wanted, so he didn't bother talking to us at all. He thought we would always say "no".

'I have no doubt that he loved us and that he knew we loved him. But love isn't enough. He thought we didn't understand him and he didn't understand us. And he was right. We didn't. He didn't.

'In today's society I'm not sure that teaching children to put others first is the right thing to do. It doesn't work if nobody else does it. I'll be telling Cathy to teach *her* little daughter to treat others kindly by all means, but to put herself first. And then, maybe for her, everything might fall into the right place.

'I would have stood up more strongly for him in the school system. I've learned that it has to be done quickly. You don't treat teachers as if they know everything, because they don't.

'I would have looked for help earlier.

'I have learned how important it is to say everything to the people we love. When my mum was dying this year I did everything I could think of to comfort her, to say goodbye. I kissed her, I thanked her, I told her how much I loved her. I said all the things that are so often left unsaid – all the things I wished I had said to Collin. In fact, I was very sorely tempted to say to her: "When you get to the other side please tell Collin I'm still bloody cranky with him".

'I didn't say it. People forget how much grandparents are hurt when young people take their own lives.

'There is something I would like to say to any young people who may be concerned about the behaviour of their friends – particularly if they know a friend has attempted suicide. They *must* tell somebody. It doesn't have to be a parent but it can't just be another mate. It must be somebody who can help.

'I read that it's better to have a friend who is now an enemy than to have a friend who is now a corpse.

'To parents, I would say: Tell your children all the good things there are about them. Tell them all the time. Make sure they know.'

'It's four years since we lost Collin,' said Jan. 'I went to the movies the other day and the people in the film were dancing. I found myself crying again. It was just so sad, remembering how happy we used to be.'

AFTER JASON

When it first happened the kids climbed into each other's beds every night so they wouldn't have to sleep alone. They dreamt about their brother all the time.

The autopsy stated that Jason Connor had died from carbon monoxide poisoning. It was stressed in the report that Jason had been an exceptionally thin man.

For nine months, Lee moved about in a fog of shock. Peter's heart, which had so much room in it for the son who was not his own, was broken. He wept often.

Lee remained stoic.

'I had to be the strong one,' she said. 'I work with families who have lost people through suicide and I knew what I was supposed to do. I had to watch out for the kids. We had lost one child through suicide and we had to make sure it never happened to us again.

'I was honest with them from the start. When they asked why Jason had died I said I didn't know. He was depressed but I didn't know why.

'Ceane was a great help. She took over everything and organised the funeral. She didn't crack until six weeks later, on Jason's birthday.'

'I still see him in my dreams,' said Ceane. 'I don't mind. That's the only way you can get to see them again, isn't it? Sometimes I can even smell him. The spot where he died has a nice view over the mountains. I often go up there and have my lunch and think about him.'

Charmaine won't talk about Jason's death.

Stacey withdrew into herself. She couldn't cry. On her eighteenth birthday, a month after Jason took his life, she realised he wouldn't be coming to see her. The family would not be together for her special day. The tears came at last.

It was her final year of high school. She studied hard because, she said, that's what Jason had always told her to do. The following year, after two months away at university, Stacey gave up her course and came home. After what had happened, she couldn't bear being separated from her family.

'Inevitably there were rumours about drugs,' said Peter. 'Erin copped a lot of flack at school. Peer pressure is very strong at that age. She took matters into her own hands. She became very aggressive. Then she tried turning the other cheek. It hasn't been easy for her at school and it's not getting any better.'

Ashleigh was brought home from the primary school several times. 'She wanted to talk about him,' said Lee. 'It did her good.

'We were very worried about Keiran. He was only six and he completely clammed up. His teachers were worried too. I arranged counselling for him at the community health centre, although he still rarely talks about Jason. If this had happened to us ten years ago, before I got into welfare work, I would not have known how to get professional help.'

'You're looking for signs all the time,' said Peter. 'We stress to the kids that if there is *anything* troubling them, anything at all, they should tell us about it. The silliest little things that don't seem important to us, can mean everything to them.

'I'm not angry any more but I still think Jason's death was a terrible waste. He had everything to look forward to. Now he won't ever get married, he won't have kids of his own, he will miss out on all of that. I'm a family man. The best thing that ever happened to me was these children of ours. And now the grandchildren are coming along. Kids are the best thing about life.'

Nine months after Jason died, Lee broke down. She lost interest in her life and children. She wanted to die. All the grit and determination with which she had fought breast cancer five years earlier, was gone. She sought professional help and leaned heavily on her husband. 'Lee got me through at the beginning,' said Peter, 'because she was so strong. By the time she broke, I was able to be strong for her.

'Being down the mines, working underground, I used to turn off the lights and sit in the dark and think about things. I used to try to talk to Jason. I told him to go and visit his mother. Somehow.'

STACEY: 'Living is harder these days. Kids want to be successful but they can't. It's too hard. It's a lot more difficult for young people to find work. Drugs and alcohol are so easily accessible. There's more pressure, both academically and socially.

'There is pressure on families too – parents take their troubles out on their children. In the fifties, children did everything their parents said; they had strong family values. Today kids can do anything. There are laws that say we can do what we like. It takes away the respect.

'We have power struggles here, we argue with Mum and Dad. But we respect them. Our arguments are always resolved.'

CEANE: 'If we don't start making things better *now* for my baby daughter's generation, it's going to be doomy to live in this world. There's poverty and the ozone layer and all those wars overseas; there's not enough money, not enough jobs, there's getting introduced to drugs and alcohol so early. There's not enough love in this world. Look at all the divorces. They happen because people give up too easily. We have to be strong enough to keep trying. Life knocks you down but you have to fight back.'

JOEL: 'I've contemplated suicide. I lost my father when I was a little kid and I lost the brother who was more like a dad to me when I was only fourteen. I've lost two close mates. You do think about escaping. But when you see the hurt it does to people, you know it's not worth it.'

LESSONS

'Nobody is interested in hearing about suicide or murder until it happens to their family,' said Peter Connor. 'Once you get involved in it, which you never do by choice, you find out a lot more about it. We heard that two of Jason's friends from school had committed suicide before he did. It didn't occur to us that Jason would try it too. You just don't think that way.

'People change gradually. You might notice something in your neighbour's family that you ignore in your own. You don't want to accept that anything is badly wrong. You're a normal family. Nothing like that happens to you.

'People should be educated to speak up about it if they notice something is wrong. Nothing could be worse, ten years down the track, than someone coming up to us and saying: "Listen, I had a feeling Jason was going to do that and I wish I'd told you, but I thought you might get upset".

'Something that really hurt us was when we put a memoriam notice in the paper on the anniversary of Jason's death. We said he had died by suicide and the editor of the local paper flatly refused to put the word suicide in. He rewrote it.

'That's the sort of prejudice you're up against. People want to hide it all the time.'

LEE: 'If only doctors took the time to explain to their patients what antidepressant medication does and how it works. If only they could arrange to have the medication followed up with the right sort of counselling.

'We need people who are already working in the community to be made aware of the dangers of suicide. Doctors of course, but also community nurses, teachers, lawyers – anybody who is dealing with people with problems. We also need qualified counsellors so they can refer troubled people to them for help.'

It's Sunday morning at the Connors' white painted brick semi in Martini Street and for a little while there's not much going on at all. Most of the older Connors are sitting around the big dining room table. Worn out with talk. Still remembering. Ceane has been crying. Lee, too, has wept a little; big silent tears trailed down her cheeks as she listened to her daughter describe the night Jason died. Ashleigh, standing behind Lee's chair, slides comforting arms around her mother's neck. It's okay, says Peter. Talking, crying, even laughing about him – it helps.

In the oven, the Sunday roast is crackling its way to its full potential. The now familiar crash of the screen door is followed by the appearance of skinny, high-speed Keiran and a small friend.

'This,' says Peter, 'is Keiran's mate, Ming.'

Lee gets up and begins cleaning off the table so it can be set for lunch. The photos are still there from yesterday. Keiran can't resist them. He stops, slows, and gazes again at the big picture of Jason.

'Who's that?' asks Ming curiously.

'My brother.'

'Your brother? Kurt?'

'No, my other brother. Jason.'

'He looks nice.'

'Yep.'

'Where is he?'

At last the Connor house is quiet. All you can hear is the snapping of roasting meat and the sibilant hiss of breaths being taken in around the table. The eyes of the adults meet; we all open our mouths to say something. There is a tightness in our throats which for a moment stops us speaking.

All of us but Keiran.

'Jason's dead,' he says.

'Gee, sorry,' says Ming.

Keiran nods and takes one more look at the photograph. Then the two little boys run out the door to play in the sun.

MORE ABOUT MA...

I've gotta tell you, being an adult is better than being a kid. Especially when your brother and sister are grown up too, and you all talk to each other about stuff you never said before and you find out they've done more than one bad thing as well; even when their bad things are not as bad as yours, you don't feel so left out.

What I found out from Edward was that Mum had a really sad life before the time she threw the spaghetti bolognaise. Her father was really strict and he belted them all with a strap if they did anything wrong – and their wrong stuff was nowhere near as bad as mine, I can tell you. Also he never treated her as well as her brothers and her mother was really quiet and never said anything, just worked herself into an early grave. The biggest surprise of all was that Mum was married for quite a few years to some guy she had fallen in love with when she was sixteen but he left her for another woman and she had to go back to live with her parents again, which was very hard for her.

I can see now why Mum would never have left Dad. She'd been dumped and alone once and she didn't want it to happen again. Also, her parents didn't approve of the marriage, so obviously she would never admit she had made a mistake. I suppose that's why she worked so hard at the perfect family image thing.

I've finally worked out why Dad cooperated with the image. He was a state ward when he was a kid and he never had a real family at all until us. I suppose nobody was ever proud of him.

ı can also understand why Mum hates men so much. She feels inferior to them. The only exception is Edward. She has always adored Edward because she made him and he never does the wrong thing.

Edward says that is not true at all. He said it's just that I have never been able to look at life from anyone else's viewpoint; he says I concoct versions of events to suit myself.

Jilly says that too – that I never considered anyone's feelings but my own. I apologised to them both. I just didn't think they were as miserable as me.

Edward says he screwed up horribly when he was young because he just opted out of family life altogether and he felt horribly guilty because he never stood up to our father. Every time he got his courage up to do it, Mum would talk him out of it. He had no idea how to rescue Jilly and me. Once he got to uni he just stayed away as much as he could.

He says I'm a terrible judge of character but he laughs when he says it and he rubs my head. We never used to touch each other much before. I wish we had done more hugging when I was little.

Quite often when I'm talking to Edward I think of that time in the car when our parents were singing together and he turned bright red. I used to think he was just dying of embarrassment. I've changed my mind now I know him better. Edward wanted so much for them to be happy. I think he was red with *longing*.

Jilly says for her whole life everyone made her feel totally stupid because she was the youngest and the plainest and not brilliant like Edward and pretty and popular and clever like me. She had to work like mad to keep up her grades and this was made more impossible by our disgustingly dysfunctional parents, not to mention my antics. That's what Jilly calls all the tragedies that happened in my life. 'The Maz Antics.' Sounds like a pop group, doesn't it?

Edward still looks exactly the same; we tell him to put mousse on his funny hair but he won't – no prizes for guessing why. But wow, you should see Jilly now. It's like those movies of plain Janes turning into ravers – she wears her hair twisted up on top of her head and she's snake-slim and she has contact lenses which make her eyes look green and enormous. She paints her lips scarlet and she always wears black and she carries a brief case. She's frantically feminist of course like all those university academics. But what would you expect, with her background?

I'm a bit of a feminist myself these days. But I still really like men, whereas I don't think Jilly does.

You know a funny thing? It was Jilly who told the principal at my school about the abortion. Isn't that a giggle? After they went to such lengths to keep her in the dark? She told the principal and Diana that it would kill our mother if she found out she had told, but she thought I needed professional help. She would have only been about thirteen at the time. It was a big favour, really, as it was their attitude which got me back into the books which is why I did so well in the HSC which is why I can still go to uni if I want to. I'm thinking about it. So I owe Jilly big time.

Danny has started ringing me again. I'm thinking about it. I suppose he can't help it if his mother is a dork.

Our father left us when Jilly left school. Mum came home from work one day and found his suitcase open on the bed. She took out some sherry glasses and the pewter mugs. Then she went and got one of the encyclopaedias and put that in instead. She knew we wouldn't be needing them any more anyway. It was the F volume, she said, in case he needed to look up fornicate when his memory gave up on him. Jilly and

I got hysterical over Mum thinking that you actually had to *remember* how to have sex.

Our father's departure has become one of our favourite family stories. We call it Dad's One Good Thing.

We all waited with baited breath for Mum to fall apart, but she didn't. She just got on with her life. As usual.

One day Edward said to me: 'Why don't you forgive Mum? It would make you feel happier.'

'She's such a hypocrite,' I said. 'All she cared about was us being a nice family.'

And Edward said: 'When you think about it, Maz, what was so terribly wrong with that?'

So I thought about it. I suppose she was only doing what she thought was best for us kids. 'She didn't come to the hospital,' I said.

'She was frightened,' Edward told me. 'Everything she had built up was falling down. She's a human being too, you know.'

I decided to forgive my mother, even though she didn't ask me to. You can't imagine what a relief it was.

I'm now supposed to forgive myself. I'm working on it.

LESSONS

When Maz announced she had volunteered to tell her story in a book about youth suicide she was surprised that her mother agreed to a brief interview. This is what Maz's mother had to say:

'Marilyn never had any intention of killing herself. She did it to draw attention to herself because she was unhappy and she thought nobody was taking enough notice of her. That's what Marilyn always did, right from the age of three.

'I haven't had a good night's sleep since the tablet incident; I'm always wondering if she will try to do it again, when things go wrong with her life. And things *will* go wrong.

Marilyn is the sort of person who attracts trauma; she seems to go from one crisis to another.

'She has always been inclined to share her problems with her friends rather than her family, although she has been closer to her brother since the incident.

'I have no regrets about trying so hard to keep my family together for all those years. Marriage is supposed to be for life. In a crisis, families stick together. People give up too easily these days. I'm not going to comment on my own situation. I'm sure Marilyn has provided lots of details. She is a great talker.

'Marilyn always wanted a lot more loving than the others. I couldn't provide enough of it to make her happy. I don't think anyone ever will, at least until she has a child of her own. That will probably settle her down.

'I worked very hard to make sure my family had everything – a nice home, nice clothes, nice holidays – I never had any of that as a child and I wanted my children to have it. Of course, my mother didn't go to work. I couldn't provide those things for my children and be at home making them happy as well although I did my best. You can't have everything, but that's another thing Marilyn didn't understand.

'I tried to do the right thing for all my family. Given another chance, and given that there are some things over which I have had no control, I don't think there is anything I would have done differently.

'The problem with a lot of kids today is that they expect to be happy all the time. Whether it's getting good marks or staying in a job – if they don't like it, if things go wrong, if it doesn't make them happy – they just give up. I suppose it's our fault. My generation turned happiness into the be-all and end-all. We should have told our children that happiness is not available whenever they want it. It's something you look forward to. It's something you hope might happen.'

'WHAT'S HOPE GOT TO DO WITH IT?'

*With all its sham, drudgery and broken dreams, it is still
a beautiful world. Be careful. Strive to be happy.*

From the *Desiderata*, found in St Paul's Church,
Baltimore, dated 1692

We had it. Our parents had it. Our grandparents had it. It
has inspired and encouraged men and women from each
generation since the beginning of time.

Hope. It is a mixture of desire, trust and expectation. It's a
desire for good and positive things to happen. It is trusting
that no matter how difficult life gets, sooner or later the bad
times will pass. It's the expectation that as time moves on, the
world will become a better place.

Hope is as essential to survival as food and water, as air, as
shelter, as love. Oh yes, love. Love is the word on everyone's
lips, love is the word on every screen's script. Love makes the
world go round.

But without hope, love is not enough.

Too many of our children have no hope. They are not as
fortunate as previous youthful generations, whose faith in a
better future equipped them to enjoy as well as endure the
turbulent years of adolescence. Young people today are
forced to fumble along without hope, struggling over the
bumpy road to maturity in their brand name joggers and

probably never even realising what a difference hope makes and how much they are missing.

They are very well-informed about the harsh realities of life. They know about stranger danger, divorce and marriage (in that order), sex, pollution, war, illegal drugs and the importance of employment before they are in double figures. Through television, beautiful picture books and magazines, we tell them everything they need to know. The argument is that this makes them better informed and more able to protect themselves than many children from previous generations, whose childhood was more sheltered and, in most cases, much more innocent.

We are neglecting our children if we don't also introduce them to beauty, truth, honesty, loyalty, obedience, compassion and kindness – the qualities of life which make hope possible.

Many people believe that this is the only generation for centuries which will inherit a world that won't be an improvement on that of their parents – that looks, in fact, as if it might be considerably worse.

How did we let this happen? How could we have been so careless and so cruel? How self-absorbed have we become that we have stolen away our children's hope and called this progress?

In our technological age, our children have more miracles at their finger tips than we ever dreamed possible. But the marvels have come at a price. We have turned today's kids into a pretty cynical bunch. Despite the lavish commercialisation in his name, they are lucky if they still believe in Santa Claus by the age of four; a falling star induces worry rather than wishing – another potential hazard to the planet. And as for rainbows! No matter how ephemeral and lovely, a rainbow doesn't need a pot of gold at the end of it any more – not when EFTPOS is available so much closer to home.

There's not a lot of hope in the newspapers or on the screens; there's not much of it in the words of our leaders, in the evidence at Royal Commissions, in the messages from our media, or in the emissions that endanger the face of our earth.

Quick, let's get some hope for the kids. Phone up. Use the Visa card. Order some hope. Take away or home delivery? Do you want garlic bread with that? Let's get some hope in *fast*.

How? We have miracle drugs and life-saving sciences, push-button food and a world-wide web of information in our schools and family rooms; but there are still no magic potions or high-tech machines which can manufacture hope and happiness.

Richard Eckersley is a Canberra based strategic analyst who has researched and written about youth issues for the past ten years. As long ago as 1988 he wrote a report for the Commission for the Future in which he analysed rising rates of youth suicide, drug abuse and crime, and the widespread social alienation and disengagement of young people. He recommended that the underlying causes be tackled.

A number of studies have found many young people to be mistrustful, cynical and fatalistic, wary of commitment, outwardly confident but inwardly insecure, alienated from society and apathetic about the future. 'They believe that life should be fast and fun; that they are on their own; that options should be kept open, governments are incapable of solving their problems and they themselves are powerless to change things,' said Richard Eckersley.

A study convened by the Australian Science Technology and Engineering Council in 1995 found that more than half of Australians aged fifteen to twenty-four thought the twenty-first century was more likely to be a time of crisis and trouble than one of peace and prosperity. Only a third thought Australia's quality of life would be better in 2010 than it is now, while a third thought it would be worse.

They acknowledged the importance of science and technology, but realised that their impact depended on who had control of them.

Their dreams for Australia were of a society that placed less emphasis on the acquisition of material wealth by individuals and competition among peers and gave a higher priority to community and family life, the environment and a society of cooperation.

This contradicts the image of adolescents as being flexible, adaptable, technologically-literate sophisticates who have learned to thrive on chaos and insecurity and are eagerly embracing the possibilities of post modern society. Most of all it contradicts the claims by so many parents that leaving kids to their own devices and taking it for granted that they will spend most of their time with their peers (rather than their family or a mixture of age groups in the community), will make them independent, capable and strong.

It also throws a shadow of doubt over the equally popular view that almost all teenagers become dreadful for a few years and then get over it; that the media focuses on extreme cases – addicts and suicides – but that these don't represent the reality.

Richard Eckersley believes most young people remain optimistic about their own lives but even this personal optimism may be crumbling under the pressures they face as they grow up and make their way in the world. Modern western culture is failing to provide them with a sense of belonging and purpose – assets which have provided previous generations and other cultures with confidence in their own worth and trust in a secure future.

The media has an enormous influence on young people's attitudes today. 'It encourages them – indeed, all of us – to live vicariously through the lives of others,' he said. 'Because of the media, we live less in our own lives now than at any other time in our history.'

Television, he says, creates public images that bear little resemblance to private realities and often focus on the trivial and the sensational. The media heighten youthful anxieties by depicting the world outside their personal experience as one of turmoil, exploitation and violence. Discontent is fuelled and self-worth eroded by promoting superficial, materialistic lifestyles and selling a way of life that is beyond the reach of most adolescents.

A youth worker in Lithgow, New South Wales, which has a disturbingly high rate of suicides in young males, strongly supported this view; no matter how hard the boys worked, he said, they went home at night to watch lives 'on the box' which were always so much more powerful, more exciting and more beautiful than their own.

The media also makes virtues of what traditionally were vices – pride, avarice, lust, envy and anger, while many traditional virtues, such as faith, charity, fortitude and above all, hope – are neglected or even disparaged.

According to Richard Eckersley, such long-established values as altruism, conformity, deference to authority and honesty, have been systematically stripped of any meaning in today's Australia.

'This doesn't mean we should return to old, traditional forms of identity and belief,' he said. 'You cannot advocate unquestioning obedience to authority if governments and authorities are leading us into further trouble.

'It does, however, indicate a serious cultural flaw. The problem for young men and women is that while the old values and traditions have been debased and destroyed, nothing has been created to take their place. There is an urgent need to broaden and deepen the meaning in their lives. In what should they believe?'

Right now the answer seems to be: themselves. It's coming from schools, universities, screens and songs. The greatest love of all is the love of self.

'Our value system emphasises the individual and his or her freedom of choice and personal fulfilment,' said Richard Eckersley. 'However, the more self-centred our values are, the poorer our relationships with others will be.'

It's all too hard. The kids want to know what society expects of them. They need responsibilities as well as rights. Too much choice leaves them floundering. If they are given only themselves to believe in, they have nothing to fall back on when things go wrong.

'It may be,' said Richard Eckersley, 'that the greatest wrong we are doing to our children is not the fractured and dysfunctional families or the scarcity of jobs, damaging though these are, but the creation of a culture that gives them nothing greater than themselves to believe in, no clear moral guidelines and no cause for hope or optimism. It is a culture whose main effects appear to be demoralisation and confusion.'

Despite this, he believes hope lies in the very fact that western society is experiencing such a profound cultural transformation.

'A new order can only emerge when an old order has failed,' he said. 'We are living in the turmoil of a profound transition in western culture but hope lies in a new beginning.'

Inevitably, a fresh start is only possible if we are prepared to recognise what is wrong and to do something about it.

There are solutions to the psychological and social problems which have resulted in the destruction of hope among many young Australians, but these solutions are not quick or simple and if they are to be effective, we all have to be involved.

After all, it's the ordinary people who want a good, caring, safe world in which to raise their families. In their book *The Making of Love*, Steve and Shaaron Biddulph suggest that out of a confusion of ideologies, politics and dogma, the world has come to a very simple turning point: 'Ordinary people ... are expressing what kind of world they want. They want an economic order which tries to be fair. They want natural beauty left in the world and freedom from toxicity in their air, water and food. They want a more human urban landscape. They abhor the cost and danger, even the *idea* of the arms race.'

Leaders who tap into the power of ordinary people can succeed by expressing on our behalf what is in the hearts of most of us. These are the leaders Australia needs. It's up to us to choose them wisely and well. But we are all responsible for the restoration of hope. The professionals and the politicians can't be expected to provide everything that's needed.

You don't need a degree in anything to show you care. To make a phone call. To take around a bunch of flowers. To write a note of encouragement. To offer a ride, a drink, a meal. To listen. To comfort. To tell a happy story. To do nothing but be there.

You don't have to be a person with religious faith to understand and practise a piece of good advice that has encouraged kindness and caring for more than 2000 years: Treat others the way you would like them to treat you.

Hope is in sharing. In good times, it's the sharing of happiness with those around us which creates the ultimate joy. In sad times, it's the sharing of sorrow which can make grief endurable; which can prevent sadness from turning into total despair. Gail Kilby, who runs suicide prevention programs for community groups, said it's easier than most people realise, to offer comfort. 'All you have to say is: "I know you are sad. I want to help you if I can." This is relevant whether you are a mother, a father, a sister or brother, a doctor, a psychologist, a nurse, a social worker, a teacher or a friend.'

Hope is with families. It's easy to be convinced by the media that the family is at the root of society's problems. The truth is that in the history of mankind, nothing has lasted so long and worked so well as a group of (usually) related people who live together and love each other. Despite all the negative statistics, a majority of Australian children are growing up in stable families.

But the family is built on sacrifice. Writing in *The Australian* newspaper in 1996, columnist B.A. Santamaria pointed out that running a family requires two people to set aside their pleasures, their opportunities and their ambitions, in order to provide for their children. 'It requires fidelity, self-discipline, economy and faith in the future.'

This would be more practically achievable in Australia if governments backed up their rhetorical support for families by creating an economical environment which made it possible and practical for one parent to bring up the children at home while the other went out to work. Prevention of problems in adolescence begins in infancy; most research continues to indicate that children benefit best from spending their early years with either their mother or with the same full-time care giver. It has been argued recently by some doctors working in the field of adolescent health that it is just as important for a parent or an adult family member to be there when teenagers are home as well.

After all, what's the point of rolling their eyes in disgust and scornfully sneering if neither Mum nor Dad is around to see it?

Until 1997, except for Medicare purposes, the existence of dependent children didn't rate a mention on an Australian income tax return.

Hope is in friendship. Many references have been made in this book to the stigma of suicide but perhaps not enough has been written about the kindness of friends. Despite their heartbreak, many families have been overwhelmed by the compassion shown not only by good friends but by people they barely know.

In times of trouble, human kindness means more than food or water or shelter or light.

Hope is closely aligned with spiritual faith. Sometimes young people need something greater than human help. For more of them than we suspect, hope may come with the belief that Someone, whomever they may conceive that Someone to be, is watching over them.

Hope is with parents who listen, friends who care and a society which offers well-trained and compassionate professionals who can listen and advise. Only when we convince them that a better world is possible will our children be able to go forward without us and make it happen.

A century ago, the French scholar, Emile Durkheim wrote in conclusion to his study of suicide: 'Once the existence of the evil is proved ... the important thing is not to draw in advance a plan anticipating everything, but rather to set resolutely to work.'

What the wise man means is – just do it.

FACING THE FUTURE

Until 1997, assistance and health care for depressed and suicidal young people and their families has been very fragmented. Not one of the many families interviewed for this book felt that they or their children had received the help, treatment, support and understanding they needed. Any assistance from health professionals and the agencies with which they were associated was haphazard and achieved largely through trial and error; hospital staff were at best kind but stressed and overworked and at worst, unsympathetic, inexperienced and impractical in the advice and treatment they handed out.

Most families who sought assistance felt helpless in the face of their unfathomable problems. Despite their own best efforts, they did not experience equitable, appropriate and efficient care.

Those lucky enough not to have been touched in some way by the death of a young person should not be deceived. Youth suicide is a more serious problem in Australian society than most of us realise. It will probably get worse before it gets better, which means a great deal more resources than have currently been made available will be needed to solve or at least alleviate the problems of young people.

In carrying out any government initiatives to achieve this goal, it will be essential for all medical and health professionals to work together.

It is also crucial that families be involved. Wherever possible, families must be consulted and included and their feelings and opinions respected, when determining the health and happiness of their children. Non-government support groups, given appropriate funding and training, have the potential to be of enormous assistance to families.

Dr David Bennett, Head of Adolescent Medicine at the New Children's Hospital, Sydney, said the problem of youth suicide would not be solved while people dealt only with the deaths.

'This is a moral issue and it confronts us all,' said Dr Bennett. 'It's at the core of what is going wrong with our society. It's proof if we need it that we have failed to provide our young people with a sense of optimism and a life that has some meaning.

'We should value and support families so much more than we do. We should value and support our young people, and listen to them. These kids who are trying to kill themselves are in trouble – layer upon layer of trouble which is not entirely of their own making. It's the responsibility of all adults who care, to do something about it.'

How will we be judged, one or two hundred years from now? Will historians report a sudden serious increase in the rate of youth suicide during the last quarter of the twentieth century, resulting from economic rationalisation policies in politics, ignorance in the community and neglect in the health system? And will they then report a marked improvement in these figures resulting from intelligent solutions and increased resources being directed at the problem?

Or will the past twenty-five years be seen as the time when a national cull of society's most vulnerable groups began by permitting young people to eliminate themselves – but only those young people who could not cope with the harsh realities of the life granted to them by the state?

As social analyst Richard Eckersley reminds us, *how well a society cares for its weak and vulnerable is a measure of how civilised it is; a society that fails to cherish its youth, fails.*

Within our families, we need to help young people develop stable, loving and loyal relationships; within our society we need to provide them with security, education, work and self-respect. Most of all, we should do what we can to give them faith in the future and the confidence to face all that life holds for them.

We must do everything we can to persuade them to stay.

EPILOGUE

The young woman lifted her flowing gipsy dress out of reach of the water and grabbing her little boy, swung him high in the air. He laughed and screamed, pummelling her plump and rosy arms with his tiny fists.

'I have to take you to Granny's so I can go to work,' she said as she settled him on her hip. 'We can come back tomorrow.'

Tears wet his eyes and he struggled and yelped, kicking his skinny legs in an effort to escape.

'Tomorrow can be something to look forward to,' she said patiently. 'The beach will still be here.'

He gouged the tears from his eyes and scowled as she put him down.

'You promise?'

'I promise.'

But he raced again into the salt-smelling sea, and looked back at her pleadingly as the spreading sheet of water once again reached for his toes.

'I've got a lot of things to do here, Mummy,' he howled. 'I just don't *want* to leave early.'

'Neither do I,' laughed Maz, catching him and hugging him tightly. 'Neither do I.'

THE NSW CENTRE FOR THE ADVANCEMENT OF ADOLESCENT HEALTH

The Department of Adolescent Medicine at the New Children's Hospital, Westmead, New South Wales, has been at the forefront of developments in the field of adolescent health and medical care for the past two decades. As well as pioneering a comprehensive, integrated and creative model of adolescent health care linking in-patient, out-patient and community services, the Department has undertaken focused research, provided undergraduate and postgraduate education and training and supported policy planning activities at both state and national levels.

The overall goal of the NSW Centre for the Advancement of Adolescent Health is to contribute to improvements in the health and well-being of adolescents and their families through:

- Better Practice Models of Health Care Delivery – developing guidelines for better practice in the delivery of health and medical care to young people and their families.

- Education and training – fostering the development of interdisciplinary education and training in adolescent and family health.

- Research Coordination – establishing a network of experienced researchers from affiliated research centres in

New South Wales to share skills and information, facilitate collaborative projects and coordinate strategic planning in adolescent health research.

- Policy Support – providing a coherent professional resource for advice on the development, implementation and monitoring of health policy impacting on the health and well-being of young people.
- Local, National and International Networking – acting as a reference point within New South Wales, Australia and internationally in it's linkage with professional bodies to ensure that professionals in New South Wales are able to contribute to and benefit from their work.

The NSW Centre for the Advancement of Adolescent Health in partnership with the Centre for Mental Health is undertaking a project which examines the barriers to young people and their families recieving appropriate mental health services and care.

A percentage of the royalties from sales of this book will go towards the Centre to fund further research into adolescent health.

THE ROSE FOUNDATION

The Rose Foundation is a non-profit organisation which has been established to:

- Reduce the suicide toll by making every community in Australia 'suicide aware'.
- Provide quality books, resources and seminars on loss, grief and suicide prevention for the community.
- Support those bereaved by suicide.
- Support sponsors to partner Rose in projects designed to *turn the tide* of suicide.

The Foundation's publishing company, Rose Education, offers a comprehensive list of carefully researched and relevant publications which are essential reading for anyone concerned with the subject of suicide prevention, awareness and bereavement. They include:

- *Hearing the Cry; Suicide Prevention* (1990) by Margaret Appleby and Margaret Condonis
- *Surviving the Pain; After Suicide* (1992) by Margaret Appleby
- *Suicide Awareness Training Manual* (1992) by Margaret Appleby with Dr Raymond King and Barry Johnson
- *Be a Friend for Life; Preventing Youth Suicide* (1992) by Margaret Appleby and Raewyn King
- *Tell Tell Tell; Preventing Youth Suicide* (1993) by Margaret Appleby and Raewyn King

- *Understanding and Helping Suicidal Children* (1994) by Margaret Appleby
- *Helping Suicidal Children; a Training Manual* (1994) by Margaret Appleby and Dr Raymond King with Barry Johnson
- *Reflections ... for those Bereaved by Suicide* (1995) Margaret Appleby and Margaret Duncan
- *Suicide Awareness for Aboriginal Communities* (1995) by Dr Raymond King, Margaret Appleby with Colleen Brown
- *Guide for the Clergy* (1996) by Gail Kilby and Margaret Appleby

WHERE TO GET HELP

The list below includes numbers for face-to-face and telephone counselling as well as numbers to contact in a crisis situation. Some of the services are just for children and adolescents; others counsel young people and their parents and families as well. Some numbers are information centres and will refer callers to the resource most appropriate for their needs.

Where the phones are manned for 24 hours, this is indicated in brackets. Other numbers are available during business hours only.

Most large public hospitals offer counselling services.

At the end of the list are numbers to ring for bereavement and support for families and friends after a suicide or attempted suicide.

ALL STATES

Lifeline (24 hours, seven days a week)
131 114 (cost of a local call)

Kids' Help Line (24 hour)
1800 55 1800 (free call)

NEW SOUTH WALES

Salvo Youth Line (24 hour)
02 9360 3000

Youth Line (a branch of Lifeline)
02 9633 3666 (24 hour)

Wayside Chapel Crisis Centre
02 9358 6577

RAPS (Resources for Adolescents and Parents)
02 9890 1500 (metro) or 1800 654 648

Parent Help Line (Centacare)
132 055

Unifam (family counselling)
02 9633 5611

The Rose Foundation (suicide prevention, counselling and community education)
02 9606 6853 (referrals to appropriate numbers in other states provided)

Relationships Australia (counselling)
02 9418 8800

NSW Association for Mental Health (referrals and advice about services)
02 9816 5688 (Sydney metro) or 1800 674 200 (country).

For government services in the telephone directory, look up health, ring the number for your own health area (there are different numbers for Sydney metropolitan, outer metropolitan and rural NSW) and ask for mental health services. In most cases you will be referred to the adolescent unit at your nearest public hospital or to a psychiatric centre in your area.

Community health centres and local crisis counselling teams can also be found in the community services section of the white pages.

VICTORIA

The Action Centre (counselling)
03 9654 4766 (metro) or 1800 013 952

Centre for Adolescent Health, Parkville
03 9345 5890

Centre for Young People's Mental Health, Parkville
03 9342 2800

Lifeworks (relationship counselling and education services)
03 9654 7360

Relationships Australia (counselling)
03 9853 5354

For government services in the telephone directory, look under health, child and adolescent psychiatric services, child and adolescent mental health services or Human Services, Department of.

SOUTH AUSTRALIA

Child and Adolescent Mental Health Services
08 8204 7389 (referrals to your nearest appropriate centre, city or country)

The Second Story Youth Health Service
08 8232 0233 (City)

08 8255 3477 (North)
08 8326 6053 (South)

Relationships Australia (counselling)
08 8223 4566

For government services in the telephone directory, look under child and adolescent mental health services.

QUEENSLAND

Parent Line
1300 30 1300 (8 a.m. to midnight, cost of a local call)

Child and Youth Mental Health Centres
07 3236 4833 (Brisbane metropolitan)

Queensland Association for Mental Health (information about services throughout the state)
07 3358 4988

Salvo Care Line
07 3831 9016 (24 hour, Brisbane metro only)

Relationships Australia (counselling)
07 3831 2005 (Brisbane metropolitan)

For government services in the telephone directory, look under Health, Queensland Department of.

Western Australia

Family Help Line
08 9221 2000 (metro) or 1800 643 000 (24 hour)

Youthlink
08 9224 1700 (metro) or 1800 803 356

PET: Psychiatric Emergency Team
08 9224 8888 (24 hour)

Crisis Care
08 9325 1111 (metro) or 1800 199 008 (24 hour)

Salvo Youth Line
08 9227 8655 (telephone counselling and referrals to appropriate agencies)

Samaritans Youth Line
08 9388 2500 (metro, 24 hour) or 1800 198 313 (country, 24 hour)

Child and Adolescent Services
08 9334 3900 (Bentley)
08 9448 5544 (Warwick)

Relationships Australia (counselling)
08 9336 2144 (Fremantle)

For government services in the telephone directory: look under mental health or children and adolescents.

Tasmania

Community Mental Health Team
03 6236 9286 (8a.m. – 10.30 p.m.) or 1800 808 890

Child and Adolescent Mental Health Services
03 6336 2867 (Launceston)
03 6233 8612 (Hobart)

Relationships Australia (counselling)
03 6231 3141

For government services in the telephone directory, look under Community and Health Services Department.

Northern Territory

RESOLVE (Anglicare)
08 8985 0000

Relationships Australia (counselling)
08 8981 6676 (metro) or 1800 652 404 (country)

For government services in the telephone directory, look under Territory Health Services and find mental health.

Australian Capital Territory

Youth Line
02 6257 2333 (4 p.m. – midnight)

CATT (Crisis Assessment and Treatment Team)
02 6205 1065 or 1800 629 354 (24 hour)

Parent Support Service
02 6278 3995

Woden Youth Centre
02 6282 3037

Relationships Australia (counselling)
02 6281 3600

INTERNET INFORMATION

Reach Out! is an on-line youth suicide prevention service catering to three specific groups: young people, family and friends and professionals. It will be available from December, 1997.

Go to   http://www.reachout.asn.au

BEREAVEMENT COUNSELLING AND SUPPORT

Club Speranza
02 9908 4574 (for referrals to support groups in each state)

The Rose Foundation (referrals to participating states provided)
02 9606 6853

The Compassionate Friends
Sydney metropolitan – 9290 2355
NSW Country only – 1800 671 621
Vic – 03 9888 4944
SA – 08 8351 0344

Qld – 07 3371 2223
WA – 08 9486 8711
Tas – 03 6243 9665

Salvation Army Bereaved by Suicide Program (NSW only)
02 9419 8695

References

Margaret Appleby and Margaret Condonis, *Hearing the cry*, Rose Education, New South Wales, 1990.

Dr David Bennett, *Growing pains*, Doubleday, Sydney, 1995.

Steve Biddulph, *Manhood*, Finch, Australia, 1995.

Steve and Shaaron Biddulph, *The making of love*, Doubleday, Australia, 1992.

Dr Sheila Clark, *After suicide: help for the bereaved*, Hill of Content, Melbourne, 1995.

Richard Eckersley, *Casualties of change: the predicament of youth in Australia*, Australian Government Publishing Services, Canberra, 1988.

Stephen J Edwards and Jon Pfaff, *Managing youth suicidal behaviour: a guide for general practitioners and community health personnel*, Commonwealth Department of Human Services and Health, 1996.

Dr Raymond King, *Trends and perspectives on suicide*, Rose Education, 1996.

NHMRC, *Depression in young people: clinical practical guidelines*, Commonwealth Department of Human Services and Health, Australia, 1997. Commonwealth of Australia, reprinted with permission.

Queensland Health, *Suicide in Queensland: suicide research and prevention program*, 1992–2.

David de Vaus, 'Suicide among young Australians' in *Family Matters*, no. 44, Australian Institute of Family Studies, Melbourne, 1996.

Youth suicide in Australia: a background monograph, Commonwealth Department of Human Services and Health, Australia, 1995.

FURTHER READING

Iris Bolton, *My son, my son*, The Bolton Press, 1986.
A first person account of a young man's death by suicide and his mother's efforts to come to terms with her own loss while counselling her family and her community.

Bronwyn Donaghy, *Anna's story*, HarperCollins*Publishers*, Sydney, 1996.
The story of schoolgirl Anna Wood's death from the drug ecstasy and an exploration of the challenges of parenting young people today.

Bronwyn Donaghy, *Keeping mum*, HarperCollins*Publishers*, Sydney, 1997.
A humorous anthology of the day-to-day business of bringing up happy children. Bereaved mother Jan Schultz has said: 'This book bought back to me all the funny and nice memories about raising our family. It made me laugh again.'

Suzanne Fabian, *The last taboo: child and adolescent suicide*, Penguin Books, Australia, 1986.
Interviews with family, friends, teachers and young people about suicide and attemped suicide.

Judith Guest, *Ordinary people*, Fontana Collins, 1977.
A novel about the relationship issues resulting from the death by suicide of one of two teenage brothers. It has also been made into a film.

Peter West, *Fathers, sons and lovers*, Finch, Australia, 1997.
Men talk about their lives – from the 1930s to today.

INDEX